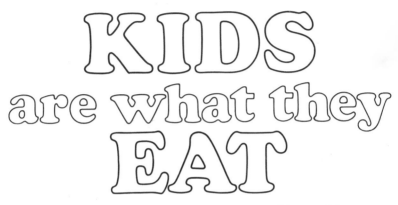

KIDS are what they EAT

What Every Parent Needs to Know About Nutrition

BETTY KAMEN
AND
SI KAMEN

ARCO PUBLISHING, INC.
NEW YORK

Dedicated

to the children of our household
KATHI, PAUL, RITA, and MICHAEL

and to our readers—
if you could see our children now, you would know what we know:
the concept of this book works!

DISCLAIMER

All of the facts in this book have been very carefully researched, and have been drawn from the most prestigious medical journals. However, in no way are any of the suggestions meant to take the place of advice given by your doctor.

Published by Arco Publishing, Inc.
215 Park Avenue South, New York, N.Y. 10003

Library of Congress Cataloging in Publication Data

Kamen, Betty.
　　Kids are what they eat.

　　Bibliography: p.
　　Includes index.
　　1. Children—Nutrition. 2. Food, Natural.
I. Kamen, Si. II. Title.
RJ206.K24 1983　613.2′088054　82–18404
ISBN 0-668-05563-4 (Cloth Edition)

Printed in the United States of America

10　9　8　7　6　5　4　3　2　1

CONTENTS

ACKNOWLEDGMENTS

Thanks to:
Michael Kamen, who finds it easy to counsel people because his insights go far beyond book-learning.
Kathi Kamen-Goldmark, who finds it easy to research other cultures because of her instinctive compassion for *all* human beings.
Perle Kinney, who finds it easy to come up with the right words any time of the day or night—just like that.
Yury Agureyev, who finds it easy to sketch cartoons because humor and joy are a natural part of his life.
Serafina Corsello, M.D., who finds it easy to share her gifted ideas because she is a great, brilliant lady.
Thanks to:
Ruth Spiegelman, Toby Pollak, and Blanche Scharfenberg for their invaluable expertise in the kitchen and their help with the references and at the typewriter.
Thanks to:
Ellen Sulzberger Straus, president of WMCA Radio, New York, for encouraging special opportunities for special causes.
Thanks to the following caring professionals:
Fima Lifshitz, M.D., Professor, Department of Pediatrics, Cornell University Medical College, New York, and Chief, Division of Endocrinology, Metabolism and Nutrition, North Shore University Hospital, New York; Warren M. Levin, M.D., Director of the World Health Medical Group, New York; Paul Yanick, Jr., Ph.D., C.C.C.A., Clinical Audiologist, pioneer in hearing/nutrition relationships; William J. Oliver, M.D., Mott Children's Hospital, Ann Arbor, Michigan; Jerome Vogel, M.D., Medical Director of New York Institute for Child Development, New York; Peter Pellett, Professor of Food Science and Nutrition, University of Massachusetts, Amherst; Ross Hume Hall, Ph.D.,

Director of En-Trophy Institute and Professor of Biochemistry, McMaster University, Canada; **Lendon Smith, M.D.**, practicing pediatrician, Portland, Oregon, and former Clinical Professor of Pediatrics, University of Oregon Medical School; **William Kaufman, Ph.D., M.D., F.A.C.P.**, pioneer in allergy/nutrition research; **Jerry Mittelman, D.D.S.**, New York, practicing preventive dentistry; **Robert Segrell**, teacher extraordinaire; **Diana Dalton, M.A.**, Counselor in Normal and Therapeutic Nutrition; **John C. Reis, Ph.D.**, Practicing Psychotherapist, San Diego; **Angel Martinez**, Youth Health Consultant and member of the Board of Directors of the National Center for Health Education; **Marjorie Marks-Katz, M.Ed., R.D.**, Pediatric Nutritionist in Pediatric Endocrinology, Metabolism and Nutrition, North Shore University Hospital.

Books are not written or promoted without editors and public relations people. We've had the *best* of both: Thanks to Madelyn Larsen and Gwen Phillips.

FOREWORD

This is a delightful book, easy to read and very persuasive for those hesitating to take the leap into health and healthful foods. All of us who have studied and taught nutrition and who have tried to get the unhealthy to adopt just a few of the concepts we are sure can improve the quality of one's life, know how difficult it is to overcome bad eating habits.

Using some clever vignettes of very real family encounters within the supermarket, Betty and Si Kamen have given us a view of ourselves and our thinly disguised self-deceptions: how we compromise and bargain with, and how we deceive our families and friends—so we may have our cola drinks, our chocolate, and our sugars! Most of us are hooked on *something*, and like the narrow-minded addict, we manipulate our whole day around getting our fix of coffee, sweets, booze, or eclairs (that's mine).

The Kamens are sympathetic and understanding with us weaklings. They are not rigid and unbending as are so many of our colleagues who insist that we all change overnight.

Betty and Si use insight therapy. They appeal to the cognitive part of our brains that can relate the symptoms and signs to particular foods, to the chemicals in processed foods, or to the sugar-laden junk that is on every shelf in every store. They are smart enough to let the reader fill in a few of the details. Readers will be able to use the "Aha! How true. Boy, that's me, all right" phrase that helps to motivate one to action. The Kamens assume the reader is bright enough to put a few things together. Now, if we can only *nourish* the cognitive part!

The Kamens' attitude of compromise is exemplified by the story of their own son who, as a young student, knew the value of whole-grain bread, but needed peer group acceptance. His sandwiches were a compromise: a slice of whole-grain bread underneath and a slice of white on top for all the world to see. He must have "played" this like a cardsharp, close to the vest. None of us wants to be too far out for fear our friends will think we are odd or, worse yet, health nuts. What Betty and Si are saying, and I can attest to this, is: slight deviations from the perfect diet are allowed at the beginning just to get someone started on the program. Feeling better or being less sick acts as its own reward and encourages continued change. It's slow but worthwhile. You have to live in that same body all your life.

My wife and I have found we survive the holidays and dinner parties by using the prefestivities C-B$_6$-calcium-protein snack. When we get to the party we are not so desperately hungry that we have to have a highball. A glass of white wine is enough to produce conviviality. We then nibble on nuts and raw vegetables that most hosts and hostesses have found keep their guests under control. When the meal is served we are mellow, and can even eat some food to which we might be sensitive. At dessert we can survive by compromising the hostess' wishes and our biochemistry. We'll eat a tablespoon of the chocolate mousse because we don't want to offend the hostess and would like to be invited again.

I hear daily from people who have gotten off sugary snacks and allergens and then could *really* tell it was bad when they reintroduced the villain.

This book is for those who have already found that diet is the key to health, as it will give them supportive evidence and insights into the mysteries of human biochemistry. Betty and Si know how to get the message through. But the book should be especially helpful to the skeptic—the one who feels that, along with the three squares a day, all we need are aspirin and Valium®.

There ought to be a law requiring that stores can only sell food that Mother Nature made. Or if the only food that could be sold would have to be approved by Betty and Si Kamen.

Thanks for a great book, Betty and Si!

—LENDON H. SMITH, M.D.

PROLOGUE

Sherry Westman, student at a junior high school in Huntington, N.Y., wrote the following composition in answer to the assignment: What would you do if you were responsible for feeding your family?

If I were responsible for my family's food, all we would eat is junk food, like pizza, hot dogs, hamburgers, french fries, potato chips, soda, and other stuff. So unless you want to be sick all the time, don't put *me* in charge of my family's food. I'm writing this because at my age all you want to eat is junk food. But when I grow up and have children, all they are going to eat is nutritional food, because I don't want to spend all my money on doctors and dentists.

Sherry has said it all. The teenagers do know, don't they?

Chapter 1

SEDUCTION IN THE SUPERMARKET

Little drops of water poured into the milk,
give the milkman's daughter lovely gowns of silk.
Little grains of sugar mingled with the sand,
make the grocer's assets swell to beat the band.
—Walt Mason, *Little Things*

Blind dates, a meeting with your child's teacher, lobster dinners, sunsets, beauty, vacations, lunch with your mother-in-law, and even sex have been evaluated on the proverbial scale of *one to ten.* Since this measurement paints a graphic picture familiar to everyone, let's examine the shopping carts of several families around the country, and classify the foods being purchased. To be certain that we are all on track, let's consider tomatoes as a case in point. Tomatoes have been developed for durability. The skin of one variety won't even crack when whacked into a brick wall at 12 miles an hour. Take this image a little further: Politicians and off-key singers will not have to be concerned with messy splattering when confronted by tomato-throwing malcontents. The politicians, the sour-note soprano, and the produce packer might give this tomato a value of *ten.* But surely the grumbling hurler would not even confer the skimpy score of *one.* What rating would *you* give these tomatoes?

Then there's the bright red apple capable of traveling to the moon and back—several times—arriving home looking as though it should take honors for prime position in a fruit bowl about to be photographed for the cover of *National Geographic.* Ten? What about:

Grains which grow quickly with artificial fertilizers
Ice cream which won't melt

Clinical Trials

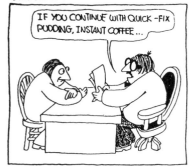

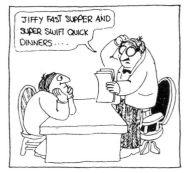

by Oldden

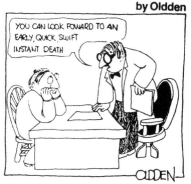

Peanut butter which doesn't have to be mixed
Salt which flows freely
Butter which doesn't have to be refrigerated
Butter which is yellow all year round
Milk in which the cream doesn't rise to the top
Potato chips which are never soggy
Bread which stays soft
Rice which doesn't stick
Rice which cooks in a minute
Mashed potatoes, which come in a box
Breaded shrimp, which are all precisely the same size
Fresh-smelling sweet cream, which is thirty days old

Obviously, we need to define our *one to ten* standard before embarking on a shopping tour. Let's not be influenced by "crispy," "pretty," "colorful," "fast," "easy," "convenient," "durable," "nonstick," or even "prestigious." Let's consider *nourishment.* Apparently the people who *grow* the food communicate with the people who *process* the food, who communicate with the people who *distribute* the food, who communicate with the people who *sell* the food. Are we asking too much if we suggest that the food grower and food processor communicate with the doctor or the nutritionist who understands human biochemistry? When and if such communication takes place, the health professional will have to define *full nourishment potential,* including the consequences in the event that such nourishment is lacking.

As with the tomatoes, that's no easy task. A piece of corn grown 300 or more years ago by American Indians was much shorter than the ears of corn with which we are familiar. But the ancient corn had more protein of better quality than today's hybrid. Do these changes suggest *demerits* or *points* for current corn crops? Suppose we disregard food quality that has been altered over the centuries (for better or worse), and judge the food as it is grown today—from the farm to the food processor to the supermarket to your table and finally to every cell in your body.

Nourishment is "that which sustains with substances necessary to life and growth."[1] *Optimal* nourishment is that which sustains with substances necessary to life and growth *in a most exemplary way.* If you put regular gas in a car designed to run on high-test, the car will run, but you'll know the difference. There's nourishment, and then there's optimal nourishment. Let's rank foods in terms of *optimal nourishment.*

A number of years ago an experiment was conducted at an aquarium. Water was synthesized. This was done to the best of the scientists' knowledge, based on what was known about the component parts of water. Fish placed in this man-made water did not survive. Perhaps some day we will know enough about water to be able to duplicate it in all its essence. Or there may always be an unknown factor—a biological phenomenon that will never be fully understood. Although scientists claim to know the chemical assay of an orange, they have yet to create an orange in the laboratory. It may be like the philosopher—forever searching for the meaning of life.

The same is true of nourishment. We know some of its complexities, and some of its processes and component parts. But we do not know nearly enough about nourishment to intercept nature and yet we produce cheese that isn't cheese (processed cheese food), raisins that aren't raisins (made from modified starch and sugar), and other synthetic foods that are nonfoods (ersatz butter, eggs, etc.). Perhaps we will be able to accept the chemists' capability to nourish us with replacement food products when they can create an orange containing seeds which, if planted, will grow into an orange tree that produces more oranges.

Dr. Ross Hume Hall, professor of biochemistry at McMaster University in Canada, suggests that viewing nutrition in terms of its parts or in terms of static numbers is a major and serious failing. By static numbers, he is alluding to the recommended dietary allowances. Nutrition, says Dr. Hall, must be viewed as a *process*. He uses this analogy:

> Eating 14 designated nutrients in a refined and fabricated food is just as ecologically unsatisfying as sitting in a theatre for three hours looking at a [still] photograph of a ballet. The phenomenon of nutrition is the phenomenon of movement.

Dr. Hall's message continues:

> The quality of health depends on the quality of nourishment.... And no one knows enough about nutrition to redesign what nature evolved.... Human nutrition is a complex biological phenomenon which is part of the phenomenon of human life.... We must seek an understanding of whole nourishment in the complete dynamic context of living processes.... The new food technology cannot change the fundamental organic nature of the eater. Food technology [does not have] at its command the wisdom to fabricate its new foods in the image of life forms that once served as human food.... Dressing a pauper in a king's clothes does not a king make.[2, 3]

A food that rates *ten* is a food that is whole and natural—a primary food—a food that has not been tampered with—a food that offers a range of nutrients, present at the time of full growth and accountable at the moment of consumption.

Let's Go Shopping!

Our supermarket extends from coast to coast. The following interviews are real. The names have been changed to protect the chocolate freaks, the sugarholics, the cola addicts, the closet health nuts, and above all the innocent. The innocent are those who are doing as well as they know how, but simply do not know how—well enough.

Family # 1

Ellen and Bob Smithers, Kansas City, Missouri
    Ellen: homemaker and part-time artist (creator of silver jewelry)
    Bob: teacher
    Children: Judy, 15; Robbie, 13; Jennifer, 10; John, 8; Sherry, 5

"But Mom, I'm having some friends over. Do you know how embarrassed I'll be when I have to say, 'Sorry, we don't have cake. We don't have soda. We don't have candy. We don't have ice cream.' My friends will never come back." Judy looked desperate as her mother ordered her to remove the packaged cupcakes from the wagon and return them to the shelf. The issue had already been discussed. Ellen Smithers responded firmly and sharply. "I spoke to Jane's mother today and Jane isn't allowed any junk foods either." "But what about the rest of the girls? How can Jane and I explain that our mothers are going through some kind of *phase?*"

    Ellen withheld a smile, and said, "I know you're angry, Judy. But this is a decision we talked about." Ellen had learned a long time ago that when she gives in intermittently, it encourages her children to whine forever. However, if she holds fast consistently, the complaints eventually peter out. As for Judy, she was having difficulty understanding why her mother wouldn't bend. Her mother was not usually so rigid about food selections, especially for parties.

    Indeed, this was the first time Ellen set limits on party fare. There were always a few restrictions on everyday meals and snacks, but the children had free rein for special events The Smithers had decided there were too many "special events" these days. Ellen had been impressed by a recent newspaper article indicting sugar. The medical study cited in the paper also pointed a finger at the high cost of these items. Not that Ellen wasn't always aware of how expensive processed snack foods are, but the *per pound* breakdown was dramatically graphic. Imagine! Potato chips are seven times more costly than bananas!

TABLE 1
SNACK FACTS: COMPARATIVE COSTS

Food	Cost per Pound
Potato chips	$2.58
Tortilla chips	2.29
French crumbcake	2.16
Fudge macaroons	2.07
Twinkies®	1.87
Grapes	1.19
Eggs	.67
Apples	.49
Fresh pineapple	.35
Bananas	.33

Costs based on items sold at King Kullen Supermarket, Huntington, New York, December 1981.

A family joke, often repeated, is: "What's the best thing Mom likes to make for dinner?" Answer: "Reservations." (Actually, for the seven Smithers, the luxury of a family meal in a restaurant is rare, especially, as Bob Smithers says, when all the stomachs in the family are "vacuum cleaners.")

With the help of at least two of the five children, Ellen does the major shopping every two weeks. She considers the shopping tour successful if the wheels of the overloaded supermarket carts all go in the same direction.

Judy was loitering in the "goodie" aisle, but her youngest brother John kept pace with his mother as she approached the packaged meat department. John was the typical "me too" sibling. He resented the fact that the school he attended mandated the purchase of lunch. Each morning, he watched with envy as his sisters and brothers scooped up their bologna, salami, or liverwurst sandwiches, and stuffed them into brown bags. The sandwiches looked and smelled so good.

Judy caught up to her mother and brother. She was carrying two bags of cookies, the bimonthly allotment. One choice was fixed: Oreos, established by unanimous decision. The second bag may vary. How-

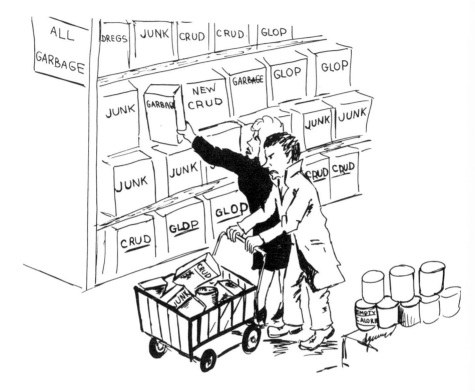

It's getting more expensive every day.

ever, Dad enjoys baking cookies, and four days after the major shopping excursion, the following scenario occurs, starting and ending the same way: "Daddy, the cookie bags are empty, and it's ten days before Mom makes her 'hit' again. Will you bake cookies for us?" Ellen intervenes. "Dad will bake cookies if you all clean up the mess afterwards." Judy: "I'll clean up." Robbie: "Of course we will." Jennifer: "Yes, yes." Sherry: "Yeah. Please." John: "Of course. Yes, yes, yeah, please." *But they never do.*

The fact that the children never clean up does not bother Ellen as much as the bribing and manipulating that takes place to get Dad to bake. However Ellen enjoys seeing her husband in the kitchen, enjoys the smell that permeates the house, and enjoys the home-baked cookies. She promises (each time) to put her foot down on the cookie issue. *But she never does.*

Before the moratorium on the ice cream, cake, candy, and soda, Ellen occasionally requested that the children hide these items from her. The children knew that this meant Mom was on a diet again. The hiding place was always the same: the refrigerator in the basement. It didn't matter that Ellen knew the secret. She was always too tired or too lazy to go downstairs anyway.

Ellen loaded the bottom of the wagon with the usual cases of cola. Bob is a cola-holic. This "corruption" is forbidden for the rest of the family, with the exception of those occasions when they dine on pizza. Then and only then do the children drink soda with their father. The double standard created by Bob's addiction is another area of deep concern for Ellen. She is at a complete loss—she doesn't know how to deal with the problem. Her best stratagem is to negotiate with the children. Her compromise: *You can have cola only when we have pizza.* Ellen knows that children learn by example, and that Bob's habit is counterproductive, both to her children's nutrition education and to her husband's health.

Cereal choices are limited to those which are not sugar-coated. Ellen reasons that the children will add their own sugar anyway. If there isn't much sugar in the cereal to begin with, the sugar intake is lessened. Obviously, the mathematics are correct, but hopefully, when Ellen learns more about nutrition, she'll know that *any* amount of refined sugar for breakfast on a daily basis is not in her children's best health interest. In addition, the lack of *fiber* in most of the boxed cereals may be as damaging as the sugar intake.

OTHERS FOOD ITEMS PURCHASED BY THE SMITHERS

Meat: mostly beef, and also pork roasts, pork chops, pork sausage
Fish: fish sticks, canned salmon, tuna fish, fresh fish once a month
Eggs: used for french toast, or served scrambled or fried in omelets
Vegetables: fresh vegetables in the summer; frozen in the winter
Fruit: canned pineapple, packed in its own juice; fresh fruit (no more canned fruit because of its high sugar content)
Nuts: Dry roasted; peanuts; yogurt-covered peanuts; peanut butter (served on crackers or white bread with grape or peach jelly)

Bread: Junk bread (Ellen's description)—white, rolls, bagels
Pancakes: Made from scratch, topped with syrup purchased in
   large can from restaurant food supplier (it's cheaper that way)
Dairy: Endless quarts of 2% milk, butter, margarine for cooking
Drinks: orange juice, frozen grape concentrate

As the Smithers left the supermarket, John said: "Some day I'll come
back and buy what *I* want."

Family #2

Pam and Frank Palmer, Woods Hole, Massachusetts
   Pam: homemaker and part-time interior designer
   Frank: accountant
   Children: Wendy, 9; Scott, 5

"Mommy, remember when you let me make the garlic soup, and I put
in three *heads* of garlic, instead of three *cloves?*" "Wendy, I'll never
forget that. And remember when you insisted on baking your first
cake alone? You were up to your elbows in dough, near tears, saying,
'It's not working. The box says *MIX BY HAND,* but maybe my hands
aren't big enough because nothing's happening.' " "Oh, Mommy, did I
really do that?"

Scott busied himself at the gumball machines while Pam and
Wendy loaded the wagon. As long as they were recalling funny
stories, Pam reminded Wendy of their visit to the automat in New
York. Wendy kept putting coins in the hard-boiled egg compartments.
After she returned with the third egg, Pam asked, "Why three eggs?
You don't even like eggs." Wendy's response was "I don't care *what* I
win!" Pam was pleased that neither Wendy nor Scott was fond of cho-
lesterol-laden eggs. The children ate eggs only once a week, concealed
in the french toast batter.

Pam and Wendy separated, covering the supermarket with the
efficiency of well-oiled machines. Wendy located the peanut butter
and the cereals (Cap'n Crunch, Cocoa Puffs, Froot Loops), while Pam
"did" the bread aisle (rye, white, bagels). Wendy headed for the
cookie section and selected the usual butter cookies (with the preserves) for herself, and the chocolate chip cookies for her brother.
Scott is a chocolate chip cookie "freak." Pam's mother-in-law sug-

gested that Pam bake cookies herself, reasoning that the cookies Scott consumed would then be of superior nutritional quality. Pam dismissed this as an old-fashioned idea that was not in accordance with her own self-image of a busy new-age interior designer. New-age women, in Pam's view, do not bake cookies.

Scott caught up to his mother and sister and triumphantly displayed his minuscule plastic prize, a horseshoe, as he chomped away on two pieces of bubble gum—the limit of comfort for his small mouth. His pockets bulged with additional pieces of gum. Scott's eye caught a package of cookies he had seen advertised on TV. He scooped the package off the shelf, and added it to the basket's bounty.

Wendy informed Pam that they needed more whipped cream, the kind that squirts from a can. "But I bought some last week." "We used it up when Susie babysat. We had peanut butter and whipped cream sandwiches."

The trio headed for the fish department. Weight-conscious Pam used very little red meat. She appreciated their proximity to the seas. It meant fresh fish any day of the year. Pam had been a heavy child and she did not want her children to have the same problem. Therefore, she eliminated red meat and also purchased fat-free milk. According to Pam, red meat and whole milk are the "fat" culprits. In addition, her reasons for rejection of these foods are intermingled with cholesterol facts and her father's early demise (heart attack, age 42). Unfortunately, there are no signs hanging in the supermarket comparing fat content of foods. Nor are there any signs explaining that once unsaturated fat is *hydrogenated,* it may be as harmful as the saturated fats.[4] Or that large quantities of unsaturated fats are also harmful.[5] Or that 9 percent of the fat in peanut butter is saturated, as is 22 percent of the fat in margarine.[6, 7]

Scott had recently gone on his first fishing trip with his Dad. He surveyed the abundance of fish with new insights, and said, pointing to the fishman behind the counter, "When I went fishing with my Daddy, we only caught one fish. I'd like to go fishing with *you.*"

There is a final stop at the soft drink aisle before checking out. Pam selected the store brand soda, thinking to herself, "It's all junk anyway. Why pay more?"

At the checkout counter Scott noticed an array of small containers on a rack, half of which were inscribed with the letter "S" and half with the letter "P." "Mommy, *my* letters. Can I have them?" Pam

TABLE 2
FAT FACTS: PAM'S PURCHASES

Food	Percentage of Fat
Margarine	80
Lamb chops	34
Peanut butter	51
Processed American cheese	30
Roasted almonds	59
Potato chips	40
Dry mix chicken noodle soup	10
Whole milk*	3½
Skim milk, 2%	2

* Not purchased by Pam, but listed to show comparison of fat content in whole milk and skim milk

From *Nutritional Value of American Foods,* Agricultural Handbook No. 454, Superintendent of Documents, U.S. Government Printing Office, Agricultural Research Service, U.S.D.A. (November 1975).

purchased a set, amused that Scott was not aware that they were salt and pepper shakers.

OTHER FOOD ITEMS PURCHASED BY THE PALMERS

Meat: lamb chops
Vegetables: frozen peas and carrots
Snack foods: roasted almonds and potato chips
Dairy: 2% skim milk; processed American cheese; margarine; fat-free yogurt with peaches and strawberry preserves; ice cream
Drinks: lemonade; cranberry juice
Sugar: small package (used only for daily cereal, ½ teaspoon each portion)
Soup: chicken noodle, dry mix

The Palmer children enjoy waiting on line to be "bagged." There are special goodies at the checkout counter, and neither Wendy nor Scott misses a single one of them.

These children offer no complaints because they have none. They get everything they want, and are more than adequately supplied

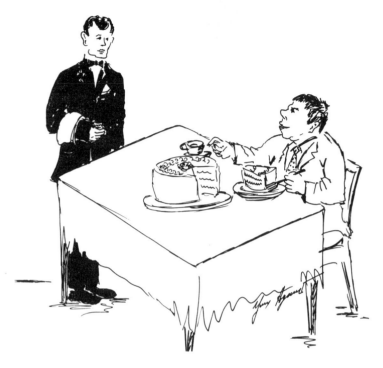

May I have skim milk for my coffee, please?

with junk food. There is never a battle when resistance is nonexistent. The behavior of their very permissive mother stems from lack of knowledge. Pam is completely ignorant of the fact that whipped cream in a squirt can is not a pure product. If it does in fact contain real cream (some do, some don't), it also contains a good deal of sugar, gasses, *and* the saturated fat which encouraged her to ban meat from her shopping list. If it is a nondairy product, it contains a potpourri of chemical additives in addition to hydrogenated oil. Pam would be confused to learn that butter and margarine have equal amounts of fat. Her awareness of good nutrition is extremely limited. Yet she *is* responding to *something.* Too bad her shoestring knowledge comes from sources that offer so much misinformation.

An interesting research effort conducted by the North American

Cultural Survey in conjunction with the Smithsonian Institute reveals
that food and nutrition knowledge of mothers of school-age children
are negatively correlated to their use of presweetened cereals: The
less the parents know about nutrition, the more presweetened cereals
they purchase.[8]

Family # 3

Nancy and Peter Harris, Tiberon, California
   Nancy: management consultant, full-time
   Peter: clothing manufacturer
   Children: Debbie, 7; Danielle, 7

Peter and Nancy exchanged glances as they overheard a mother say to
her young son, "If you don't touch anything, you can have whatever
you want." The use of food for behavior control is almost universal,
but the Harrises are trying hard not to perpetuate the practice. They
are critical of anyone who does.
   As the Harris family passed through the bakery department, the
baker emerged with a tray of hot rolls. He offered them to Debbie and
Danielle. The twins refused the rolls. They had just come from the
Chinese restaurant, a weekly treat that preceded the Friday-night
shopping tour. Peter Harris is an incessant tease and prankster. In a
stage whisper, his eyes twinkling, he prodded his daughters: "Take the
rolls. Take the rolls. *I* want them." The fact is, he wasn't teasing, and
his daughters knew it.
   The message that Peter is imparting to his daughters has to be
confusing. Obviously, Peter is not entirely sold on "good nutrition."
   Perhaps he does "believe," but is still screaming out for the
"bad" foods, which is not unlike an addict looking for a fix. His mis-
directed humor (or deep-rooted feelings) is another aspect of the difficulties of imprinting good eating habits on children: Peter is fostering
the hypocrisy of the aphorism "Do as I say and not as I do." The girls,
well-schooled in teasing techniques, often ask their Dad what he eats
when he's alone.
   In the cereal section Debbie and Danielle try to get their parents
to purchase at least one box of Count Chocula. "Please, please, pretty

please." "I'll clean my room for a week." "I'll eat salads for a month." "I'll take baths without being told for a year."

Peter said, "Listen girls, when Mommy isn't around, we'll go to a restaurant for the good stuff." Nancy flashed an annoyed look. "Just kidding, just kidding," said Peter. The girls knew from the start it was "no go." Despite the fact that the Harrises joke about the importance of nutrition, the ground rules have been set, but they play the game anyway. As they walked away with the usual purchase of raisin bran, Debbie said, with an attitude of having won a debate, "I saw my teacher eat a Twinkie last week." Danielle added in a loud voice, attempting to embarrass her parents, "How come we have junk food only when company comes?"

As Peter and Nancy selected the fresh fruits and vegetables, the girls wandered off. They returned, all giggles, asking, "Can we have this? Read the label. You'll see it's okay." On the front of the box of noodles were the words "U.S. Recommended Daily Allowance, RDA %: Protein, 10%, Thiamin, 35%, etc., etc." On the back of the box, the all-revealing small print had been ripped away. The girls knew that every time the small print was read, the package was promptly re-

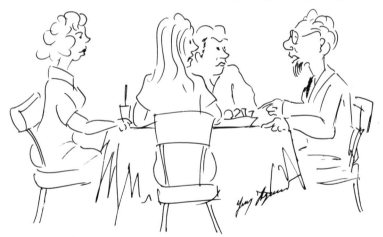

It's aluminum calcium silicate with a pinch of isobutylene-isopyrene cipolymer. But today we added methyl valerate in your honor. Hope you like it.

turned to the shelf. They mischievously tore off the information that condemned the noodles. They also knew their parents would see through their trick, and as they returned the package to the shelf, they said, "Can't we have it anyway—just this once?" Before the sentence was completed, the noodles were in place.

A few last pitches were made before checkout time. Debbie: "My friend Jonathan says his mother wouldn't have cartons and cartons of soda in the basement if soda was poison, like you say it is." Danielle: "If I can have the ice cream, I'll take my vitamins twice." Debbie: "We'll brush our teeth right after we eat it."

OTHER FOOD ITEMS PURCHASED BY THE HARRISES

Meat: lamb, veal
Fowl: chicken
Fish: fresh fish; canned tuna
Bread: whole wheat, sourdough
Vegetables: all fresh, variety
Nuts: natural peanut butter
Snack Foods: cheese, Häagen-Dazs; dry roasted nuts
Dairy: whole milk, yogurt with fruit, cottage cheese, sour cream, butter
Drinks: frozen orange juice, canned grapefruit juice, apple juice
Soup: canned, used as base for leftovers
(Sugar is kept on hand only to cure hiccoughs or to place on itchy mosquito bites.)

As the groceries were being tallied, Danielle appeared with a cereal box that had a game printed on it. "We'll throw the cereal away and use the box."

Somehow, some way, when the Harrises arrived home, there was a package of doughnuts in one of the bags. What began as a pleasant family ritual turned out to be a power struggle. The Harrises' strength in handling the twins' food requests are in contradiction to their attitude concerning the children's behavior, and also to the messages the children receive from their father. Perhaps the dichotomy stems from the fact that the selection of healthful foods is new for the Harris family. There is still a degree of artificiality involved in the total implementation of good nutrition for the whole family. And children see through this—better than adults.

TABLE 3
THE LARGE PRINT GIVETH:
THE SMALL PRINT TAKETH AWAY

Food: Frozen Fried Chicken Dinner

INGREDIENT LISTING, FRONT OF PACKAGE, LARGE PRINT:

Fried Chicken, White Portions; Mixed Vegetables in Seasoned Sauce, Apple Cake Cobbler

INGREDIENT LISTING: SIDE OR BACK OF PACKAGE, SMALL PRINT:

Chicken breast portions with back portion (fried in vegetable oil), reconstituted dehydrated potatoes, water, enriched wheat flour, peas, carrots, corn, reconstituted whole milk, rehydrated apples, margarine, sugar, salt, vegetable shortening, dextrose, vegetable oil, modified food starch, soy flour, sodium phosphates, eggs, apple concentrate, monosodium glutamate, algin, apple powder, leavening, spice, vanilla extract, whey powder, natural flavoring, and citric acid

Food: Noodle Roni Romanoff

INGREDIENT LISTING, FRONT OF PACKAGE, LARGE PRINT:

Egg noodles, cheddar cheese and sour cream sauce with other natural flavors

INGREDIENT LISTING: SIDE OR BACK OF PACKAGE, SMALL PRINT:

Enriched egg noodles with niacin, iron (ferrous sulfate), thiamine mono-nitrate, riboflavin, cheddar cheese, salt, amioca starch, nonfat milk, dried onion, natural flavors, partially hydrogenated vegetable oil (contains one or more of the following: cottonseed oil, palm oil, soybean oil), dried garlic, lactic acid, citric acid, artificial color, FD&C yellow No. 5.

Food: King Vitamin

INGREDIENT LISTING, FRONT OF PACKAGE, LARGE PRINT:

A Corn and Oat Multi-Vitamin and Iron Supplemental Cereal

INGREDIENT LISTING: SIDE OR BACK OF PACKAGE, SMALL PRINT:

Corn flour, sugar, oat flour, salt, rice flour, coconut oil, brown sugar, sodium ascorbate (a vitamin C source), vitamin E acetate, reduced iron, niacinamide (one of the B vitamins), FD&C Yellow No. 5, margarine [partially hydrogenated soybean oil, liquid soybean oil, partially hydrogenated cottonseed oil, cultured skim milk and skim milk, salt, mono and diglycerides, lecithin, sodium benzoate (a preservative), artificial flavor, beta carotene, vitamin A palmitate], FD&C yellow No. 6, pyridoxine hydrochloride (one of the B vitamins), riboflavin, thiamine mononitrate, vitamin A palmitate, folic acid, vitamin D_2, vitamin B_{12}.

Family # 4

Helen and Roy Garcia, Baltimore, Maryland
Helen: housewife
Roy: cabinet maker
Children: Paul, 12; Lisa, 8

"Mommy, when I was a little girl we used to buy food like that. How come?" "Honey, we found out we had been making a mistake. We just didn't know any better." Helen's response was straight from the shoulder, as honest as can be. She was not uncomfortable admitting her errors. She hoped her children would understand that one is never too old to learn and improve. Helen saw no reason to be defensive.

As Helen and the children selected their sprouted whole-grain bread, Paul asked a special favor of his mother. "Mom, can we find a loaf of white bread that isn't too junky? I feel funny being the only one of the guys eating such dark bread." Helen agreed without hesitation. Paul had come a long way from the early days, when the Garcias first initiated food changes. At that time, Paul expressed total disdain. After his scorn, he entered a stage of purposefully grabbing any food item he knew his parents would reject. And if he ever caught *them* buying canned food or eating other contraband, they'd never hear the end of it: When Paul discovered a box of fancy cookies that had been purchased for a dinner guest, he tacked a note on the package reading, "I hope you feel guilty when you eat this."

Now Paul seeks food which meet with their approval. Sometimes his concept of what is sanctioned and what is taboo is slightly distorted. For example, heavy advertising and peer pressure have convinced him that frozen pizza is totally acceptable. But it had been a long time since Paul accused his mother of child abuse. He no longer asks "Why can't I—everyone else does." Helen decided that if adolescent sensitivity could be protected with a variety of bread that isn't totally healthful, why not? She was empathic regarding peer pressure, recognizing that Paul's desire to be "one of the guys" was appropriate at this age. She also knew that Paul's chances of being seriously teased by his friends were slim. Children are not always democratic or respectful of individual differences, but annoying ridicule is so often the result of aggressive behavior—unrelated to the tease-target. Paul was popular, and his friends were an especially nice group of boys.

Helen vividly remembered Paul's first concession to the values of good food. They were sitting at the dinner table one day, the sun streaming in on Paul's face. "Your complexion is superb, Paul. How lucky you are." "Ah, gee, it's probably all that garbage you make me eat."

Lisa, encouraged by her brother's success with the white bread, attempted to get on the bandwagon. She held up a candy bar. "We never, never have this. Just this once—and we won't tell Daddy, okay?" "I tell you what," answered Helen, "how would you like to select the ingredients for your birthday cake today? Anything you like." Helen had a homemade cake in mind, a cake baked from scratch. But Lisa conferred much more status on a stir-and-bake ready-mix.

Helen knew she had blundered as soon as she uttered the words "anything you like." She could have given Lisa specific choices. Her attendance at parent effectiveness courses proved very helpful in cop-

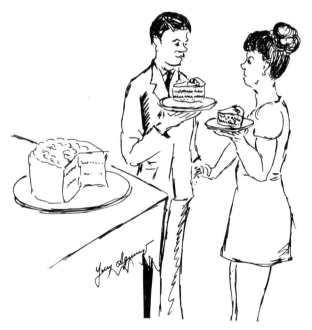

It's just like mother used to make. She was a chemist.

ing with food transition issues. Each time she erred, she gained more and more insight. Helen had learned that explicit, clear-cut limits are easier for children. Ambiguous restrictions are as confusing as *no* checkpoints at all. Children need boundaries that are in accordance with the values of the family. They want to know their parents care enough to set the parameters.

As she thought about it later, Helen also knew she should not have avoided Lisa's petition for candy by diverting attention to the birthday cake. She was simply substituting one junk food for another. She could have said, "We've already planned for one treat. Let's make that selection. Your choice for a birthday cake can be a carob cake or a cheesecake. We'll bake it together. Let's purchase the ingredients for the cake now."

OTHER FOOD ITEMS PURCHASED BY THE GARCIAS

Meat: none
Fish: fresh only
Fowl: whole fresh chicken
Vegetables: fresh, variety
Fruit: fresh (variety), lots of apples and bananas
Nuts: Trail Mix
Cereal: Cheerios, shredded wheat
Snacks: health-style corn chips, sesame bars (Protein-Aide)
Dairy: yogurt (plain), butter, buttermilk, eggs
Drinks: apple juice
Soups: none (soups are homemade)

At the checkout counter, the Garcias met Connie, the mother of one of Paul's close friends. Pointing to the contents in her wagon, Connie looked a little embarrassed. "We're having a big bash this weekend," she apologized, because of a conversation she and Helen had a few days earlier. Helen had called the mothers in Paul's scout troop to discuss snack contributions. Each parent, and especially Connie, "talked it up" when confronted with the subject of nutrition. Each claimed to run junk-free kitchens. Helen sensed if she checked their refrigerators at that moment, she would find the very foods they denied serving. But Helen knew the women weren't lying. Many parents really believed they were limiting negative foods, or thought it was

TABLE 4
A CAKE BY ANY OTHER NAME IS *NOT* THE SAME

Style of Chocolate Cake	*Ingredients*
HOMEBAKED CAROB RAISIN CLUSTERS	⅓ cup warm water; ½ cup milk; ½ cup sifted carob; 2 tablespoons butter; 2 tablespoons lecithin granules; 1 cup peanuts; 1 cup raisins
HOMEBAKED SOUR CREAM CAROB CAKE	½ cup butter; 1 cup honey; ¾ cup carob; 1 cup water; 1¾ cups whole-wheat pastry flour; ½ teaspoon salt; ½ teaspoon soda; ½ cup sour cream; 1 teaspoon vanilla; 3 egg whites
STORE-BOUGHT PEPPERIDGE FARM CHOCOLATE FUDGE LAYER CAKE	Sugar, partially hydrogenated vegetable shortening (soybean, cottonseed, palm and palm kernel oils), bleached wheat flour, corn syrup, water, whole eggs, cocoa processed with alkali (dutched), chocolate liquor contains 2% or less of each of the following: dextrose, leavening (baking soda, baking powder containing sodium acid pyrophosphate, cornstarch, monocalcium phosphate, calcium phosphate), modified food starch, mono- and diglycerides (emulsifier from hydrogenated vegetable oil), dextrin, salt, propylene glycol monoesters, gelatin, polyglycerol esters (emulsifier from hydrogenated vegetable oil), sodium caseinate, lactylic stearate, ethoxylated mono- and diglycerides, natural flavor, xanthan gum, lecithin
DUNCAN HINES SWISS CHOCOLATE DELUXE 2 CAKE MIX	Sugar, and dextrose, enriched bleached flour, vegetable shortening (partially hydrogenated soybean oil), dutched cocoa (processed with alkali to enhance flavor), leavening (baking soda, dicalcium phosphate, monocalcium phosphate) to make cake rise, propylene glycol monoesters (for smooth texture), modified food starch, salt, artificial flavor, mono- and diglycerides (for smooth texture), cellulose gum (for smooth batter)

okay to serve some of them as long as the dinner meal included vegetables.

Whatever the reason, Helen noticed that most of the mothers "boast big" about healthful eating, but do not follow through in practice.

Family #5

Shirley and Tom Davis, Woodbury, New York
Shirley: photojournalist, full-time
Tom: lawyer
Children: Amy, 6; Linda, 1½

"Hi, Gerry. How are you?" Tom met a neighbor in the frozen food aisle. "I'd be a lot better if Becky wasn't with me." Gerry chased after his two-year-old and, catching her, held her firmly so that he could chat with Tom. "Oh, I know what you mean. We're so happy Linda isn't walking yet," answered Tom, pointing to Linda, a captive of the supermarket wagon seat. "As soon as she becomes independently mobile, no more trips to the supermarket with her."

"But Linda and Amy are such placid children. Not like my perpetual-motion machine here." "Gerry, calm or active, they get you. When Amy sat in the wagon, she couldn't see the bottom shelves. When she was old enough to walk, she demanded everything she saw at her eye level. That's where all the candy and junk foods are—the items advertised on TV. The marketing people are very clever. Amy went around singing every commercial song. As soon as she was a little older, we taught her to distinguish between junk food and good food. In fact, at age three, she went up to another child and said, 'How come your daddy lets you eat that? It has preservatives.' If we told her she couldn't have something, she said, 'I guess this has a lot of sugar, right?' Or, 'Is this bad for me? I don't want it.' We heard her advising her friends: 'Don't you know if you eat junk food you become a pile of junk?' We thought we had it made.

"Then Amy reached her fourth birthday, Linda was born, Shirley went back to work, and all hell broke loose. She pounded our heads in until we bought this or that junk food. She even threw temper tantrums for food she didn't like. 'But I'll eat it, I promise,' she would yell. Or she would scream, 'I'll buy it with my own money.' Four years old! Now we take turns shopping at night and we just don't take her anymore."

"Thanks, friend, you're giving me a lot of encouragement." "But that's the way it is, Gerry. And let me warn you. The main bone of contention is the breakfast cereal."

Tom opened a freezer door and selected a package of preservative-free ice cream. "These upright freezers stock the ice cream in full view. It was easier when the food was in deep chests. And here's the rest of the bad news. Don't ever send your child shopping with the grandparents. They are totally permissive. If the grandchild picks up half of what is in the market, the grandparent would pay for every bit of it."

As though choreographed with precision synchronization, a child went dancing after a gray-haired gentleman, calling out, "Please, please, please." Grandpa turned around and said softly, "Yes, darling." Tom and his friend laughed. *"Please* is the most frequently heard word uttered by children in the supermarket."

OTHER FOOD ITEMS PURCHASED BY THE DAVISES

Meat: hamburger patties

Fish: snapper, blue fish (fresh), canned tuna

Fowl: chicken parts

Vegetables: fresh (variety)

Fruit: fresh (variety)

Nuts: assorted (in the shell), sometimes shelled nuts purchased at the natural food store, peanut butter (natural brands, served with honey)

Cereals: Cheerios, Grape Nuts, Wheatena, oatmeal, Puffed Rice

Bread: whole-wheat (preservative-free)

Cake: Ingredients for home baking, including chocolate chip cookies, which is a family weakness

Snacks: sugarless lollypops, salted whole-wheat pretzels

Dairy: low fat and skim milk, packaged cheese (Cheddar, Swiss, cottage, and cream), mayonnaise, low-fat yogurt with flavor or fruit

Beverages: frozen orange juice, apple juice

Beans: refried beans (canned), chili (canned)

Grains: brown rice or Uncle Ben's converted

TABLE 5
CEREALS: MAYHEM IN THE A.M.

Cereal	% of Sugar	Cereal	% of Sugar
All Bran	14.0	Lucky Charms	50.4
Alpen	3.8	100% Natural with	
Alpha Bits	40.3	apples & cinna-	
Apple Jacks	55.0	mon	17.2
Boo Berry	45.7	Pep	14.0
Bran Buds	25.0	Pink Panther	49.2
Buc Wheats	13.6	Post Toasties	4.1
Cap'n Crunch	40.0	Product 19	4.1
Cheerios	2.2	Puffed Rice	2.4
Cinnamon Crunch	50.3	Puffed Wheat	3.5
Cocoa Krispies	45.9	Quisp	44.9
Concentrate	11.0	Raisin Bran	
Cocoa Puffs	43.0	(Kellogg)	21.0
Corn Chex	7.5	Raisin Bran	
Corn Flakes		(Skinner)	9.6
(Kellogg)	7.0	Rice Chex	8.5
Corn Flakes (Kroger)	5.1	Rice Krispies	11.0
Count Chocula	44.2	Shredded Wheat	2.0
Country Morning	25.0	Shredded Wheat	
Crunch Berries	43.4	spoon-size	2.0
40% Bran	16.2	Sir Grapefellow	40.7
Frankenberry	44.0	Special K	7.0
Froot Loops	53.0	Sugar Frosted	
Frosted Flakes	44.0	Corn Flakes	15.6
Frosted Mini		Sugar Frosted Flakes	42.0
Wheats	28.0	Sugar Pops	39.0
Fruity Pebbles	33.6	Sugar Smacks	56.0
Frosted Rice	39.0	Super Sugar Crisp	40.7
Grape Nuts Flakes	3.3	Team Flakes	14.6
Grape Nuts	6.6	Total	8.1
Heartland	23.1	Trix	46.6
Honeycombs	48.8	Vanilly Crunch	45.8
King Vitamin	21.4	Wheat Chex	2.6
Life	14.5	Wheaties	4.7

Percentages calculated by: Center for Science in the Public Interest, Washington, D.C.; *Brand Name Guide to Sugar*, Nelson-Hall, 1977; *The Good Food Compendium*, Doubleday, 1981.

As Tom scooped up the grocery bundles and Linda, the baby spied a box of Apple Jacks on the next checkout counter. Linda, at age 1½, sang her very first tune: "Appa-Ja . . . Appa-Ja . . ." (and whatever the rest of the words are).

Family #6

Irene Barron (divorced), Fort Lee, New Jersey
  Irene: teacher
  Children: Susie, 6½; David, 8

Unwrapped balls of soap were on display in a wicker basket. Susie fingered the pretty little colored rounds with affection. "Sorry, honey," said Irene kindly, "You know that's too costly. A large cake of soap will leave only *one* remnant to discard. Those little fellows are wasteful.'"

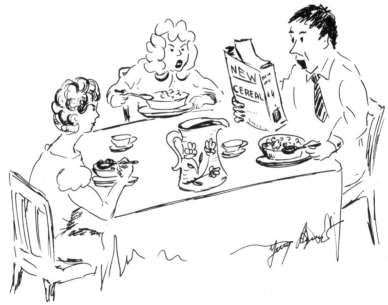

Look. This one actually has some cereal in it.

Irene greeted three of her neighbors walking down the aisle. They had carpooled to save gas, and were shopping with newspaper clippings and coupons in hand. "No—don't get the canned peas here. They are cheaper at King Mart. We'll go there next." Irene would have liked to be in on the money-saving junket to three supermarkets, but time was at a premium. She had to do the best she could in one quick trip, limited funds notwithstanding.

A more favored desire of Irene's is to shop in a natural food store. That's out of the question—a fantasy. The supermarket is cheaper than any small store, health-oriented or not. That's Irene's view.

In rapid order, Irene selected the items on her list: the largest loaf of preservative-free whole-wheat bread; one box of shredded wheat and one box of Cheerios; a huge bottle of salad oil; a few large cans of generic-labeled canned vegetables; several packages of

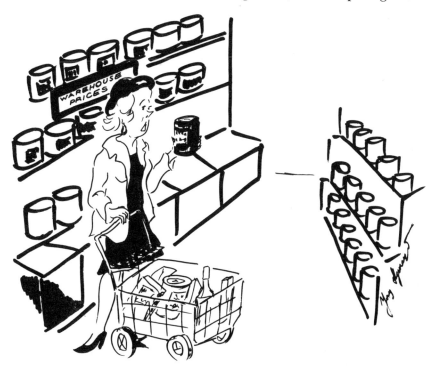

At these prices, they should *gild* it, not can it.

TABLE 6
CHICKEN: "SUM" OF ITS PARTS

Type of Chicken	Cost per Pound
Whole fresh chicken	$ .79
Chicken breasts, whole	1.49
Chicken breasts, split	1.59
Thighs	1.19
Wings	.79
Parts, frozen and breaded	2.16

Costs based on King Kullen Supermarket, Huntington, New York, December 1981.

chicken parts; hamburger meat; a few boxes of pasta, and, for those dog-days, the emergency K-rations: frozen TV chicken dinners.

Irene hesitated at the paper goods section. A package of 350 napkins saves money, but she couldn't stretch today's food budget to include this item. She scanned the boxes of rice. "Minute" is easy, but Irene knew that anything "instant" or "quick" or "prepared" is more costly. She finally selected Carolina enriched. It was the cheapest.

Roughly computing the cost of her purchases, Irene concluded that she had enough money for a package of ready-grown alfalfa sprouts.

TABLE 7
VEGETABLES: THE COST OF PRESERVATION

Vegetable	Canned (price per pound)	Frozen (price per pound)	Fresh (price per pound)
Broccoli	$	$1.74	$.69
Carrots	.59	.58	.33
Green beans	.85	1.76	.69
Potatoes	.55	.92	.19
Zucchini		.95	.69

Costs based on items sold at King Kullen Supermarket, Huntington, New York, December 1981.

TABLE 8
DINNER: THE COST OF CONVENIENCE

Meal	Cost per Person
Frozen Chicken Dinner	$1.55
Chicken	
(quartered from whole, fresh chicken)	.80
Oriental Rice	
(brown rice with stir-fried vegetables)	.40

Costs based on items sold at King Kullen Supermarket, Huntington, New York, December 1981.

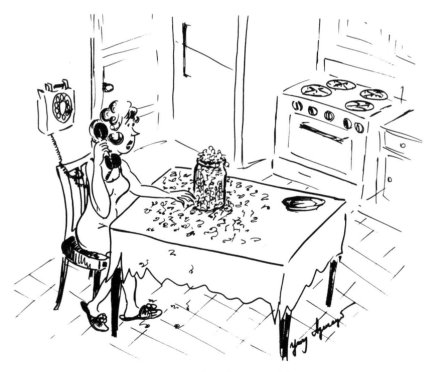

Two *teaspoons?* I thought you said two cups!

TABLE 9
RICE NUTRIENTS: FOUND AND LOST

Nutrient	Brown Rice (mg per 100 grams)	Milled Rice (mg per 100 grams)	Percentage of Loss
Thiamin	0.34	0.07	80
Riboflavin	0.05	0.03	40
Niacin	4.7	1.6	65
Pyridoxine	1.03	0.45	57
Pantothenic acid	1.5	0.75	50
Inositol	119.0	10.0	92
Choline	112.0	59.0	47

From Robert S. Harris and Endel Karmas, *Nutritional Evaluation of Food Processing,* second ed. (Westport, Conn.: AVI Publishing Co., 1977), p. 151.

Susie was still playing with the soap when Irene entered the checkout line. It was difficult enough for Irene to make healthful selections in a marketplace full of tempting high-calorie, nutritionally deprived foods. Watching the budget so carefully compounded the pressure. Irene wished she could have purchased the pretty soap for Susie.

TABLE 10
NICE RICE HAS THE RIGHT PRICE

Type of Rice	Cost per Pound
Brown (nonorganic)	$ .89
Brown (organic)	1.13
White, enriched	.57
Minute	1.82
Converted	.93
Boil-in-bag	1.36
Frozen Italian	1.44
Frozen Oriental	1.74

Costs based on items sold at King Kullen Supermarket, Huntington, New York, January 1982.

TABLE 11
ARITHMETIC LESSON

1 pound of alfalfa sprouts, ready-grown		$2.75
Cost of alfalfa seed	$2.62 per pound	
To yield 1 pound of sprouts, use 6 table-spoons of seed		.30
Savings for homegrown sprouts		$2.45

Family # 7

Beth and Victor Chapman, Burbank, California
  Beth: freelance writer
  Victor: computer consultant
  Children: Liz, 5; Michael, 2

Beth purchased one carrot for Liz and wiped it off as best she could. On occasion it was an apple—but it was always something chewy. The distraction worked. Liz never asked for pretzels or candy in the supermarket.

    Beth couldn't resist checking out the contents of other people's wagons. Although she was almost compulsive about it, she made her observations unobtrusively, and did not go to extremes, as her mother did. Beth's mom followed through with lectures to young parents whose purchases were not to her liking. When Beth scolded her about this practice, her mother quoted William Wordsworth, saying, "The best portion of a good man's life has to do with acts of kindness and of love." "But, Mom," Beth would quickly respond, "Kipling tells us 'meddling with another man's folly is always thankless work.' "

    As usual, there were no surprises. Most of the baskets were laden with foods that would never appear on Beth's own shopping list. Because there was such a paucity of fresh vegetables in the general selections, Beth often joked about starting a national organization for the prevention of vegetable extinction. She would call it "The Society for the Preservation of Parsley." Beth's purpose in being in this marketplace was the need to replenish the family's supply of paper napkins—and other necessary products from that same department.

Liz struck up a conversation with another five-year-old, which led to an exchange between the two mothers. The women chatted about growing opposition to the opening of a fast-food restaurant on the corner of a suburban street (an issue that had received widespread publicity); about TV restrictions for children; junk food restrictions for children; and about school lunch programs. From the overtones, an observer would ascertain that they were concerned parents, but no one would guess that each was an ardent "health food" devotee. However, the rapport and vibrations between the women were keenly felt, and finally, somewhat timidly, Beth said, "I notice you too are shopping for paper goods. Aren't you food marketing today?" And the cat was out of the bag.

Beth had often observed that although many parents claim to serve healthful foods, the *purists* (and she was one of them) rarely discussed their maverick food regimen, which is so out of kilter with the rest of the world. She, and others like her, broached the subject with caution, if at all.

Now kindred souls, the women shared information:

Who has the best chickens?
How do you know they are free-running?
Did you hear that Doctor So-and-So had been harassed because he
        treated arthritic patients with niacin?
What kind of yogurt starter do you use?
Do your children take brewer's yeast?
Do they swallow tablets?
Do you sweeten your oatmeal cookies? With what?
Do you give your children vegetable juices?
Where do you get good quality nuts—in the shell?
Do you have a source for goat's milk cheese?
Did you ever have luck making sauerkraut?
How do you feel about milk for the children? Wheat?
What is your favorite millet recipe?
If you want very good buttermilk, go South on Route 101 to Smith's
        Farm. Knock on the door to the left and say, "Beth sent me."

After exchanging phone numbers, Beth's new friend offered an anecdote. "A few months ago we received letters from school advising us about a kidnapping spree in our neighborhood. Children were being lured into a car with the offer of candy. My children said, 'Candy! If anyone offered us that junk, we'd run the *other* way.' Obviously, the message was not being received in the context intended. We had to start again, and state categorically, 'DON'T GO INTO A CAR WITH A STRANGER NO MATTER WHAT,' whereupon my seven-year-old said, 'I know. Not even if someone offers me watermelon.' "

○ ○ ○

Before leaving the supermarket, let's drop in on the express lanes, where a few quick trips are in progress.

Family: The Camerons, Staten Island, New York
Selections: Devil Dogs, Ring Dings, canned fruit cocktail, Rice Krispies
Comments (from 13-year-old Heather): "Mom, do you see this pimple on my nose? I'm never, never, never going to eat junk food again—starting next week."

Family: Laura Longman (divorced), Urbana, Illinois
Selections: roasted peanuts, farina, Honey Nut Flakes, brown sugar, yogurt
Comments: None. Laura shops alone. She discovered she spends from ten to twenty dollars more when her children accompany her. It's cheaper to hire a babysitter.

Family: The Calabrisis, Houston, Texas
Selections: pasta, broccoli, eggs
Comments (from 15-year-old Brian): "What! No green peppers? Just because they're expensive! You're forcing me into green pepper withdrawal."

Family: The Millers, Troy, Michigan
Selections: canned orange juice, Cream of Wheat, whole-wheat bread, skim milk
Comments (from six-year-old Sarah, holding processed cheese spread): "But it's *cheese*—isn't that good?"

Family: The Murrays, South Hadley, Massachusetts
Selections: bananas, buckwheat cereal, sprouted-wheat bread, flounder
Comments (from five-year-old Holly, upon being offered a lollypop by

a well-intentioned lady on the checkout line): "No, thank you. That's too good for me." "No, no," whispered her father. "You're supposed to say, 'I'm too good for that.' "

Family: The Olsens, Pineville, Missouri
Selections: fresh vegetables, shredded wheat, brown rice, yogurt
Comments (from seven-year-old Kate): "Since you've been listening to that nutrition lady on the radio, we never get anything good anymore."

Family: The Glassers, Tucson, Arizona
Selections: Fritos, potato chips, soda, popcorn
Comment (from Mrs. Glasser): Michelle, when you have your party this afternoon, I refuse to get involved. I don't want to watch this junk being consumed. I'm going into my room, door closed, with a good book."

Family: The Randolphs, Hollywood, Florida
Selections: skim milk, pita pouches, canned tuna, juices in containers
Comments (from ten-year-old Mollie): "But this gum is *sugarless!* Why can't I have it?"

Family: The Smiths, Phoenix, Arizona
Selections: frozen vegetables, skim milk, cheese, cup cakes
Comments (from five-year-old John, pointing to a box of cereal): "I need all that good energy, Mom." John's mother responded, "Oh, no you don't. You already have too much energy." But she purchased the cereal anyway.

We have eavesdropped on Supermarket, U.S.A. Getting back to the *one to ten* gauge, we noted many scores of *two* or *three*. *Four* and *five* popped up here and there. A rare, but occasional *ten* surfaced. If we pooled the entire collection—if we were looking for an *average*—for one great big nationwide supermarket shopping basket, the benchmark would certainly be at the low end of *full nourishment potential.*

The power of merchandising, the power of packaging artistry, the power of convenience, the power of television, the power of peer pressure, and the power of product placement are all difficult weap-

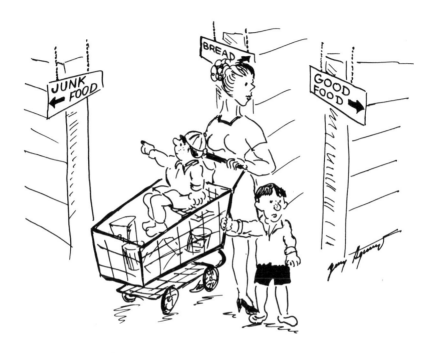

ons to combat. As we "listen" in, we get the feeling that almost everyone is trying. Everyone knows the identity of the real junk foods. A simple apology or rationalization follows their purchase. Most people think they know which foods are more healthful. There are a few food items that people are confused about. And no wonder. Even the experts can't seem to agree. The Surgeon General has said:

> Although evidence keeps mounting that certain food factors and current dietary habits may be linked with health problems as diverse as heart disease, tooth decay, obesity and some types of cancer, consumers often find it difficult to make informed choices about food.

And that's what this book is all about. It's a guide to help you make informed choices for your children—a guide about food, but not without consideration for feelings.

Chapter 2

COPING IN THE SUPERMARKET

They brought Daniel, and cast him into the den of lions.
—Daniel, VI, 16

How will Ellen Smithers ease the tension created between her and Judy? What will Judy's friends say when they learn there is no candy, cake, soda, or ice cream at her party? Will Wendy and Scott grow up to be fat adults? Will the Harris twins ever stop fooling around in the supermarket? How long will Peter Harris' "gut" scream out for the foods he used to eat? Will Paul Garcia ever go back to eating whole-wheat bread when lunching with friends? Will Linda Davis be allowed back in the marketplace? Will Susie Barron still be eyeing pretty soap when she's a teenager? Can Irene's fantasy of shopping in health food stores become reality? Have Beth and her new friend created unrealistic worlds for their children because of their stringent good-health practices? Will their children rebel later on?

Yes, the questions do have soap-opera overtones (which is not so farfetched: a recent survey reveals that nutrition ranks second only to sex in terms of people's current interest). After all, food does speak a language: food can show that you belong. Food can offer solace. It can define an occasion or a season. It is a tool for interpersonal communication. The necessity to eat motivates people to "get together," just as "getting together" justifies eating. Nathaniel Hawthorne in *The House of Seven Gables* comments that "life, within doors, has few pleasanter prospects than a neatly arranged and well-provisioned breakfast table."[1] Food is all these things. *But is it always nutritious?*

As a result of our visit to Supermarket, U.S.A., two facts surface:

1) **There is a growing awareness of nutrition.**
2) **There is a growing frustration in implementing food changes.**

Why the weak link between nutrition enlightenment and diet conversions? The attempt at food changes within a family may reveal the strength of the family unit. If you have a wholesome family structure with good relationships, the strain, if any, will be minimal. When parents have a high self-regard, children admire their parents and emulate them. That's how boys learn to become men and girls learn to become women. The best way to influence your children is to lead good, passionate, dramatic, creative, respectful, and loving lives. Your children will have wonderful role models, and you won't have to sit down and tell them how to live. This applies whether the issue is religion, politics, or nutrition. Children with this kind of background go out into the world with bright eyes, and they in turn try to see how to "do it right." Everyone thinks it's so cute to watch birds teaching their young to fly. It's not only cute, it's vital. Parents teach best by example too!

If you are parents of very young children, nutrition changeover is easy. A six-month-old doesn't make choices. But as children grow older, *they* must learn to do the discriminating. A five-year-old should have more discretion than a three-year-old, and a ten-year-old more than a five-year-old. Many parents know intuitively not to expect more than a child is capable of at various ranges of growth. (Piaget's intellectual development stages serve as an excellent guide to understanding children's capacity for various types of judgment. See Appendix for additional information.)

If you are making sudden changes when your child is fifteen, it is unlikely that your teenager will be entirely cooperative. You have probably thought about the changes for awhile, and have come to the process of change through a process of thinking. Your decisions to alter food habits didn't just happen, and it's really *your* journey. In your child's view, it's as though you were going along at 90 miles an hour, and suddenly slammed on the brakes—and there are no seat belts. Pow! At the same time that you are saying, "Don't do it," the media and the culture are saying, "Do it. It's important. It's even sexy."

You want your children to grow up in as perfect an environment as possible. In that sense, each of you will fail because your children will be touched by so many below-par shots—so many defects—in the many worlds that they will be grazing in, worlds they will coexist in, hand to hand, worlds that *do not include you.* Your values of food and nutrition may be solidified, but you need to have an appreciation for the fact that your children are going to be imperfectly nourished—not only emotionally and spiritually, but physically—by the rest of the world. You, however, have outranking influence.

Dr. John Reis, noted psychotherapist of San Diego, dislikes the negative connotation of peer *pressure.* "It would help," explains Dr. Reis, "if we called it peer *influence.*" He adds:

It is essential for children to be influenced by their peers. From the time children are born, they and their parents struggle with the separation process, frequently until the children are in their middle twenties or older. It is largely through the influence of friends and peers that children learn to develop a separate identity from their parents and their family.

Although the struggles of a teenager with personal and social identity and peer influence may appear destructive (and sometimes it is destructive), it is a critical part of growing up. At the same time, it's important for you to be aware of your own stake in influencing your children, protecting them, and preventing them from being corrupted by the outside world. The more secure you are with yourself and your spouse, the more your children will assimilate your values. But there is (and ought to be) a limit to the control you have once your children get outside of the home.

Differentiating themselves from you, and establishing a unique identity for themselves, requires that your children actively question and test your values. It should help you stay relaxed and oriented if you can experience this nonviolent rebellion as a creative maturational adventure, rather than an attempt to thwart your authority and values.

Children need stability and gradual development even more than you do. Therefore, new concepts in food should be introduced slowly, with you doing most of the initial explorations yourself, without too much imposition on the children. Encourage the children to join you in your exploration, but realize that it is your expedition. Your world and your child's world do not always coincide. So introducing changes gradually, even if done awkwardly, can be an effective way of making your children partners and avoiding taking a rigid self-righteous posture in introducing changes in your family.[2]

With some of these concepts in mind, let's look at the scenarios described in Chapter 1.

Family # 1—The Smithers

SUMMARY

Ellen Smithers has gained a new consciousness concerning the importance of nutrition. She is trying to apply the knowledge swiftly. However, she has impinged on her daughter's sense of freedom. Judy wants to have junk food at her party, food she is accustomed to serving. Her mother is vetoing a few specific items (candy, cake, soda, ice cream) because they are full of sugar. Sugar seems to be the first target of Ellen's recently acquired "new" nutrition awareness. Her actions are in sharp contrast to her husband's cola addiction, and even to some of her other purchases. Cold cuts, for example, offer severe nutritional insults.

JUDY'S PARTY

As commendable as Ellen's efforts may be, it would be less confusing if she understood the full spectrum of food change and of good nutrition before embarking on serious lifestyle modifications. We are living in a world in which many are slowly gaining knowledge of nutrition, but there is a danger of people not fully understanding all the concepts involved. Dr. Serafina Corsello, renowned director of the Huntington, New York, Stress Center, says:

> Unless we train ourselves to understand and look at the nutrition problem in the Gestalt concept of mind and body together, we are going to alienate our children. We must also acknowledge that our country has made very many mistakes in departing from natural nutrition. This is of prime importance for the evolution of the total acceptance of improved eating habits for the new generation.[3]

Ellen's rigid stand is confusing Judy. Judy is sincere when she states that she is ashamed of revealing her mother's "born-again nutrition phase." *She* recognizes that her mother does not understand the entire concept. Judy is also at an age characterized by a tremendous need to be emancipated from the constraints of her parents. Because of this strong adolescent breaking-away pattern, peer influence is of great significance in Judy's life at this time.[4]

Of course, as a parent, you are in authority. You are in a position to set the limits. Your children do not have to agree with the curbs, but the burden of deciding on limitations is *yours*, not *theirs* (until they are older). In other words, it's not the children's responsibility to reject your limits, but it is your responsibility to listen to their feelings about the limits you have set. After giving them audience, you may decide that some boundaries may be negotiated, but others can't be changed. (A non-negotiable restraint would be: no milk for a milk-intolerant child who gets stomach aches from milk exposure. Frequent consumption of milk for such a child slowly undermines health.) Whatever the resolutions, they should be clearly aired with the children.

The discussion in the supermarket between Ellen and Judy indicates that the issue had not really been talked through thoroughly. Again, there's nothing wrong with saying, "No more," and again, it is helpful to understand that your children will feel uncomfortable with your new ideas. If special treats are occurring too often, you can work out a plan to stay within acceptable limits, such as "so many times a week, or a month." However, if the decision is an unqualified *no more,* then that's what has to be presented to the children. They will be angry, as Ellen wisely sensed. This is to be expected. The next step is to find a safe way of dealing with the anger. Allow the older children to express that anger; allow them to talk about their feelings, and *listen to them.* Allow them to be grumpy. You might even say, as Ellen did, "I know you are angry, and that's okay."

New modes of behavior are being set, and these are in collision with very basic needs. It hurts to give up these needs. The matter becomes an emotional one, and for younger children it may help to offer more physical outlets. One family we know produced a play and invited friends. In the play, the Yogurt Monster was kidnapped by the Broccoli Burglar, and both the Sugar Queen and Captain Cake came to the rescue. You could make models of nutrition charts or health food stores and allow the younger children to smash them, or even throw missiles at parent models. While the limits and the goals are in transition, outlets and empathy are a necessity.

◦　　◦　　◦

The conflict between Ellen and Judy may not have been avoided completely, but if Ellen had clarified her stand at home, she would not have to assume such an authoritarian role, saying "Yes," "No," "Put it back." Working out agreements often avoids deadlocks. When children's needs and thoughts are respected, they'll respect your limits. (That doesn't mean they won't complain.)

Surprisingly, children come up with solutions you may never have considered. When you "hear" your children and take their wants seriously, they'll be amazingly creative about solving problems. One young lady developed an international pita party with the help of her mother and a close friend. She printed a large sign saying "POISON," which she placed over the candy-soda-cake tray. The group arranged a large basket of pita pouches which they surrounded with bowls of Mexican chili, Indian chicken curry, spicy Italian meatballs, Greek lamb chunks with raisins, and American health salad. The girl's friends ignored the "poison" display, and devoured the ethnic food. The international theme gave the hostess clearance for serving healthful foods with no apologies.

Since this is a beginning of change for the Smithers, it might have been less detrimental if Ellen had not held firm at this point. Or, perhaps Judy could have had the option of two of the four sugar offenders, or she herself could have come up with additional healthful (but delicious) desserts. There would have to be a great deal of trust between Judy and Ellen (going both ways) for *Ellen* to offer party suggestions which would be acceptable to Judy. Ellen would have to be in touch with what teenagers find suitable. The better way? Let the children do the planning, within the family's disciplines.

Some of the same principles are applicable for younger children. Instead of stating categorically, "We cannot have this because it's bad," allow the child to select among choices. If your goal is long-term effectiveness, it is better to start by *adding*, rather than *taking away*. A "hands-on" party works well for the younger set. This requires the participation of the guests.

Although these ideas solve many problems, be prepared to labor a bit more than usual for their execution. They are worth the effort. Don't *buy* a party for your children; encourage them to create one, or, if the children are young, create one with them.

DAD'S COOKIES

One of the difficulties encountered during the food change process is that there are often other power struggles going on at the same time. For example, the Smithers' cookie "deal" is more than a nutritional affair. How effective is the cookie allotment when the children know they can always fall back on Dad's home-baked goodies? The issue is one of lack of parental clarity or limits, and misuse of dessert. It is perfectly acceptable to make an agreement at the outset of a plan, but everyone has to meet the responsibility of carrying through. Although food should never be used as a reward for clean-up, it is appropriate to ask the children to clean the counter before the baking begins, or to wash the baking pans at the end of the project. If they don't meet their obligations, why not leave the baking pans dirty (stick them in the freezer to avoid spoilage), so that next time around it's twice as hard to get ready? The children should accept the responsibility for the natural consequences of what they are doing (or not doing).

Food is a very nurturing substance. How nice that Dad bakes!

DAD'S COLA

Children feel victimized when faced with parents who do not present a united front. Ellen is fully aware that her husband's cola addiction is undermining her efforts. It has to detract from the good and positive habits that she is trying to inculcate. This, unfortunately, is a common problem: Many children do not find their parents in unified agreement or practice. The best you can do is talk about it openly. As adults, we understand that for some people, the longer a food habit is practiced, the more resistant to change that habit becomes. You begin to respond like Pavlov's dog, with conditioned behavior.[5] However, the children do not want to hear that it is easy for *them* to change habits because they are young, but difficult for their parents. It's a hard nut to crack. Michael Kamen, our education consultant, offers this advice to parents:

> Eventually, children need to make decisions for themselves. There are choices throughout life. The best way to make wise choices is to be given opportunities to make choices. The more choices you are confronted with as you are growing up, *the better you become at choosing.*

TABLE 12
THE COOKIE MONSTER (IT DOESN'T HAVE TO BE):
INGREDIENTS OF PEANUT BUTTER COOKIES

HOMEMADE (GOOD GUYS)	½ cup unrefined oil; 1 cup peanut butter (organic); ½ teaspoon sea salt; ½ cup whole-wheat pastry flour; ½ cup raisins, 1½ cups water
HOMEMADE (BAD GUYS)	1½ cups white flour; 1½ teaspoons baking powder; ½ teaspoon salt; ½ cup margarine; 1 teaspoon vanilla extract; ½ cup sugar; ⅓ cup corn syrup; 1 egg; 1 cup commercial peanut butter
STORE-BOUGHT (GOOD GUYS)	100% whole-wheat flour; pure creamery butter; pure honey; rolled oats; unsulfured molasses; whey powder; wheat germ meal; pure vanilla; baking soda; cream of tartar
STORE-BOUGHT (BAD GUYS)	Enriched flour; sugar; brown sugar; peanut butter (which contains peanuts, dextrose, mono-glycerides, salt, sugar), lard (and may contain hydrogenated beef fat, soybean, cottonseed, or palm oils); peanut butter chips (which contain sugar, hydrogenated modified palm kernel oil, dried whey, peanut butter, cocoa, artificial flavor); sodium acid pyrophosphate; sodium bicarbonate; calcium sulfate; corn starch; monocalcium phosphate; calcium stearoyl-2-lactylate; dried whole egg; dried whey; salt

Allowing children to make choices does not mean that there are no limits or that there are no responsibilities. Quite the contrary: Children for whom clear limits are set are better able to handle responsibility.

Is it acceptable to restrict the children's cola consumption while dad indulges? Different families may have discrepant values. But the decision—whatever it is—is not as important as making that resolution *clear*. The family's specific values should determine the limits.

The determinations may be:

1) You children have no choice; you may not have cola; 2) It's okay for you to have cola once a week (or once a month); 3) As a

parent, I own my responsibility not to allow the cola but you own your responsibility and may buy the cola with your personal money.

It is possible to alter the amount of cola consumption as the entire family evolves in its nutrition understanding. Or you may know enough now to decide that you never want to be responsible for giving your child cola. (You'll probably come to that decision by the time your reach Chapter 7 of this book.) Don't get yourself into trouble by making rules that are not enforceable, or asking children to do things that are inappropriate for their age. Don't say, "You will not have cola in the outside world," but say, "I worry about you drinking cola." Children will test your limits, and will be confused if you have set limits which you do not enforce. The important thing is to be clear about your standards and to allow choices wherever possible, within the limits of those values. If, in your good judgment, you have decided not to offer any choices for cola, be certain to allow food choices in other matters, such as meal planning, etc.[6]

Another area of difficulty stems from divergent views of divorced parents. One child stated that she figured out there was no Santa Claus when her stocking at Mom's house was filled with chocolate goodies, and the stocking at Dad's contained oat cakes and carob bars. 'Santa Claus wouldn't do that to me,' she thought. Then she realized Dad was the health advocate.

A very interesting study shows that when there is disagreement between husbands and wives concerning food served at home, it's the women who are more likely to give in.[7] However, when the health of any family member is threatened, other family members will be influenced favorably—they will all eat foods beneficial to the ill person.[8]

If Ellen Smithers could induce her husband to visit a reliable medical nutritionist for his next routine physical checkup, the chances are that Bob will discover that the cola and other food insults are taking their toll. Medical nutritionists are expert in predicting the course of disease, and encouraging *prevention.* Bob Smithers might be threatened enough to cancel his cola requests.

The Society for the North American Cultural Survey informs us that younger children drink more nutritional beverages than older children, probably because the younger ones haven't had as much exposure to the non-nutritional substances. They don't have as much control over their own food intake. Milk and fruit juices generally give way to cola, which increases in popularity with age. The fact that cola contains caffeine, an addictive drug, adds fuel to the flame: the more you drink, the more you crave. *However, there is a decrease in cola consumption upon education.* Learning the effects of cola consumption has its impact.[9]

Mrs. Smithers could engage the children in a project to educate their father. They can all research and clip articles on the dangers of cola drinks. An effective way of accomplishing this goal is to present small bits of information daily. In addition to educating Dad about the deleterious effects of the cola drinks, Dad will know his children care about him. At the same time, it is a learning experience for the children. However, for this plan to be successful, the children must want to do it.

THE CEREALS

Ellen herself contributes to double standards when she forbids the purchase of sugared cereal, and then permits the children to add sugar to the cereal. Many parents who have similar viewpoints have different levels of tolerance when it comes to manipulating the diet. Some parents tell us they allow sugar to be added to cereals just as the Smithers do. Others buy sugar-coated cereals, and do not sanction the additional sugar. Still others select those brands with the least amount of sugar. But sugar is sugar is sugar—whether added to the cereal, or whether it's part and parcel of it. Since budgeting is an important aspect of large family living, perhaps Ellen will learn that boxed cereals are extremely costly compared to home preparation of sugarless cold

TABLE 13
BEVERAGE BALLOT

1960	Milk	Coffee	Beer	Soft Drinks	Tea	Juice
	37.9%	35.7%	15.1%	12.3%	5.6%	2.7%
1978	Soft Drinks	Milk	Coffee	Beer	Tea	Juice
	36.0%	25.0%	24.0%	23.0%	12.0%	4.0%
1990	Soft Drinks	Beer	Milk	Coffee	Tea	Juice
(Projection)	50.1%	27.6%	17.5%	16.7%	16.5%	5.0%

or hot cereals. (See recipes for cereals in recipe section.) In addition to fabulous taste and increased nutrients, the homemade varieties provide *fiber*—helpful to children who tend to constipation and/or allergies.

Family # 2—The Palmers

SUMMARY

Pam is permissive. Her choices in the supermarket are not varied. She restricts egg use, but allows unlimited consumption of sweets. Son Scott is addicted to chocolate chip cookies. The children have wide berth when it comes to junk foods. Pam uses skim milk; does not eat meat.

TABLE 14
CEREAL: AGAINST THE GRAIN

Cereal	Cost per Pound
Cocoa Puffs	$2.09
Dinky Donuts	2.02
Froot Loops	1.91
Special-K	1.76
Alpha Bits	1.76
Cheerios	1.68
Rice Krispies	1.65
Shredded Wheat (spoon-size)	1.45
Unsweetened Granola (natural variety)	.95
Homemade Granola: You can put it together yourself at far less cost than any of the above (*see* recipe section).	

Costs of commercial cereals based on prices at King Kullen Market, Huntington, New York, December 1981.

Cost of natural granola based on 5-pound package available from Walnut Acres, Penns Creek, Pennsylvania. (See resource list in Appendix.) Ingredients are: oat flakes, rye flakes, oat flour, peanut oil, apple juice, raisins, almonds, natural vanilla extender, cinnamon.

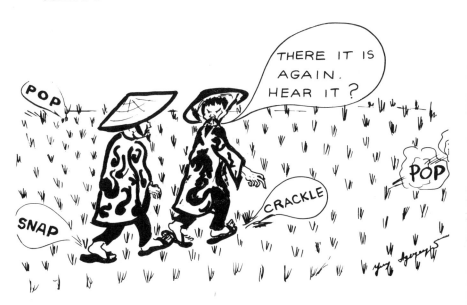

NUTRITION EDUCATION

When people know what to do, do they do it? Do most people assume they know what to do? Pam does not appear confused. She simply does not have enough information. What would encourage Pam to change the contents of her shopping basket? The answer is: More education. Countless nutrition books flood the market, obviously to little avail. The books are sold mainly in natural food stores. People who shop in natural food stores are already turned on to better eating habits. Therefore, these books reach a very select audience. Selling nutrition books in supermarkets would be in conflict with too many products on their shelves. But the supermarkets are not villains. Any store will sell the kind of commodities its customers request. More healthful items will be available in the large marketplace if and when people demand them. Do you think we can ever woo the food industry executives to join you and your neighbor in the nutrition education process?

It has been demonstrated that *classes* are the most efficient way of helping people make changes.[10] (We hope this book will be more helpful because we are dealing with specific issues of changing food customs.)

Wendy and Scott appear to be bright children, which may intensify attempts at food alterations because of their mother's permissiveness. As stated in *Nutrition, Behavior, and Change:*

> . . . children [make] use of some of the emotional meanings of food which they have learned—knowledge they have acquired through the manner in which the [first stage of the] problem was handled. One of the emotional challenges in growing up is learning how and when to assert one's individuality effectively. A bright child quickly learns that he has a tool for exerting power over a well-meaning but unwise mother by his *eating behavior.*[11] [Italics ours.]

Children are successful in getting their parents to make purchases of their choice about forty-five percent of the time.[12] We can view this statistic either as the optimist (the cup is half full) or the pessimist (the cup is half empty). Let's be totally positive: If fifty-five percent of parents can resist being manipulated by their children, *you can do it too!*

PAM'S PERMISSIVENESS

Although Pam's knowledge of nutrition is limited, she gives us the impression that she follows rules when she knows what the rules are. Is it possible for her to be so completely unaware of the dangers of excesses of candies and cookies for young children? Or has she found permissiveness an easy way out? Is she confused about how to set limits? Or does she consider herself a loving mother by "giving in"? Pam should understand that there are better ways of demonstrating love for a child than allowing excessive consumption of cookies and candy.

PAM'S LIMITED FOOD SELECTIONS

Pam typifies the "limited-food-selection" American family. A major threat to health has been developing slowly in this country because of the lack of variety in food options. The range of food preferences has narrowed considerably. In fact, 80 percent of children's food choices can be coded in only seven categories. Responses to preferences get *narrower* as the children get older. In other words, as the youth of

America age, they prefer a more limited number of main dishes for dinner. From a nutritional standpoint, this is not desirable. One reason this is happening may be the proliferation of pizza parlors, hamburger shops, and steakhouses. There is simply no exposure to a greater variety of foods. The restaurants narrow the choices of food.[13]

It is unfortunate that children do not react against "sameness" in food as adults do.[14] In addition to the self-imposed desire for restricted food choices, two other factors are stumbling blocks:

1) *Television.* Young children are exposed to about 13,000 commercials for food in one year, but these are only for 80 or 90 products, representing less than *10* product categories.[15]

2) *Loss of variety in farming systems.* Today's agriculture concentrates on corn, wheat, and soy beans which, together with sugar, sup-

TABLE 15
FOOD CHOICES: GROWING PANGS

Order of Preference	Ages 3 to 5 Food Choices	Ages 6 to 8 Food Choices	Ages 9 to 15 Food Choices
1	Peanut Butter and Jelly Sandwich	Peanut Butter and Jelly Sandwich	Cola or Soda
2	Cereal	Cereal	Cereal
3	S Milk	Cola or Soda	Peanut Butter and Jelly Sandwich
4	a m e Cola or Soda	Milk	Pizza
5	Orange Juice	Pizza	Pie
6	Pie	Fruit Juice (not Orange)	Milk

VEGETABLE CHOICES			
1	Carrots	Corn	Corn
2	Corn	Carrots	Carrots
3	Beans	Beans	Beans

Ary J. Lamme III and Linda Leonard Lamme, "Children's Food Preferences," *The Journal of School Health* 50 (September 1980): 398–399.

ply about 75 percent of the calories consumed in North America. According to Dr. Ross Hume Hall:

> North American consumers have fallen into the trap of this one-dimensional thinking. . . . They go through life unaware of the wealth of variety denied them.[16]

So what's a parent to do? One answer: the more occasions your children have to encounter different foods in diverse conditions (especially as their food habits are being established), the more easily will they accept unfamiliar foods later on. In addition, repeated exposure to new foods creates an atmosphere of familiarity with that food in due time.

THE EGGS

Despite the fact that the average American family has curtailed its egg consumption, United States children have higher cholesterol levels than children in most countries.[17] There is overwhelming evidence of the benefits of eggs. Among the reports:

☆ Dr. Eva Snead of San Antonio, Texas, describes eggs as being marvelously protective against toxic substances. "Being the most perfect protein and being most similar to human protein," says Dr. Snead, "eggs absorb toxic substances. This means they bind—not chemically, but physically—in such a way that they sludge the toxins off and make them pass through our intestines without being absorbed into our blood stream."[18]

☆ Eggs are an excellent source of complete protein. They contain all essential amino acids (one large egg contains 7 or 8 grams of first-class protein). Also found in eggs: vitamins A, B_2, D, E, niacin, copper, iron, and phosphorus. The egg yolk contains the richest known source of choline found in lecithin—necessary for keeping the cholesterol within the egg emulsified. The egg yolk also contains biotin, one of the B-complex vitamins.[19]

☆ Eggs are the only substantial source of [natural] vitamin D eaten regularly by children.[20]

☆ Because a small package must guarantee development of the young animal without recourse to outside sources of nourishment, eggs are fairly concentrated sources of the nutrients particularly essential for growth. Thus a chicken egg provides vitamin A, iron, and protein of the highest quality.[21]

☆ Egg yolks contain ... lecithin, an unusual fat-like compound which has the special property of being able to dissolve cholesterol and other fats.[22]

☆ The egg is one of the few foods that can't be tampered with before it reaches us, because it comes in its own container. The sulfur contained in the egg (the mineral which turns your silver spoon black) is required by our bodies daily, and not readily available in other foods.[23]

☆ Eggs have the essential amino acids in balance closest to that necessary for human beings.[24]

Unless Pam recognizes the error of her ways, the Palmer children may be denied this inexpensive, nutrient-dense food for the rest of their lives. Dietary patterns of childhood are so often carried throughout life.[25]

THE PEANUT BUTTER

Wendy's preference for peanut butter is not unique (see Table 15). A mother of three very young children said, "I'll know I've 'arrived' when all my kids are old enough to eat peanut butter and jelly sandwiches for lunch. How easy it will be then!" Peanut butter and jelly is almost universally given to younger children because of its low cost, easy preparation, and nutrient value.[26] More parents give the peanut butter sandwich more credit for good nutrition than it deserves. At least you have half a chance if the peanut butter is freshly ground from whole nuts and packaged without additives and sugar.

Adding whipped cream to the peanut butter sandwich could be an acceptable special treat, but not when the chemicalized variety of cream is used. Whatever happened to real whipped cream?

THE COOKIES

At the first session of the 95th Congress, it was stated by Dr. Jay Tepperman at the *Council on Children, Media and Merchandising* that:

> Food is taken for [hedonistic] purposes for pleasure, and this is something that happens very early in childhood, which I think is a sad thing. The children very early in life begin to associate the ingestion of sweet food with pleasure.... At that age in child-

hood it is possible to develop eating habits which can become very deleterious later in life.[27]

The big mystery, as yet unexplained, is: why the sweet tooth, which is universal and time-honored. Our ancestors satisfied their sweet tooth by eating fruit. Dr. Rudolph Ballentine theorizes that sweet fruit is nature's enticement: People eat the fruit and carry the seed to deposit elsewhere and propagate the growth and spread of the plant species. He states that by concentrating sugars around their seeds, the fruit-bearing plants are able to please the palate and successfully compete for attention. The sweet taste is the bait to get you to do nature's work.[28]

We've come a long way from propagating plants when we satisfy our sweet tooth today. We are inundated with foods that provide very little, if any, nutritional value, but are palate-pleasers. We no longer select our foods for the sole purpose of filling our stomachs. Industry has isolated the essence of sweetness, adding it to a wide range of al-leged edibles. People rapidly develop a craving for refined sugar—yet there is absolutely no physiological need for it.[29]

The cookies that both Wendy and Scott prefer could be made at home with healthful ingredients. There is no reason that a child can-not have a nourishing cookie. Today, many women do not consider food preparation the creative adventure it once was. However, since concern for health is often the most important influence in changing food selections,[30] it is entirely possible that Pam would either bake cookies or find a source for a more healthful brand. But for such moti-vation, she needs to be more nutrition-aware. Pam may choose not to

TABLE 16
WHIPPING IT UP: EXERCISING YOUR THUMB OR YOUR ARM

Style of Cream	Ingredients
Homemade Whipped Cream	Heavy sweet cream
Reddi-Wip	Pasteurized and homogenized cream, nonfat milk solids, sugar, corn syrup, mono- and diglyc-erides, artificial flavor, whipping gas—nitrous oxide

go back into the kitchen, which, as she sees it, is diametrically opposed to her lifestyle. But she can find ways of feeding her children properly without sacrificing another human being—namely herself. Parents need to face the commitment they are making *together*, and accept the fact that if there are children, this will limit each partner's total freedom. The solution does not have to be in fast-food permissiveness. This is child neglect—from ignorance, not malice.

Scott's chocolate cookie addiction portends trouble. Dr. Serafina Corsello comments:

> This type of addiction in childhood could make Scott a candidate for further addictions. He may go from chocolate to coffee, and perhaps escalate from coffee to other stimulants. Once the body is accustomed to stimulants such as the methyl xanthines (found in chocolate), there are risks. It is a nutritional-psychological-sociological involvement. You can see the handwriting on the wall. This is the child who may become so stimulant-dependent that he may ultimately wind up with the drugs on the street.
>
> Another aspect of the problem is the TV imprinting. The child sees the cookies advertised and wants them. The only way to protect your children from the negative advertising on TV is to make the children aware that they—and we—are being brainwashed. Raise their level of consciousness as to what is really happening. It is essential to do this because children are not only more vulnerable to the toxic substances, but also to the toxic ideas. To counteract brainwashing, you need education. And you can educate your children from early years on.[31]

THE FISH

Pam's extensive use of fish is typical of those who lack an understanding of the complexities of the necessity to rotate foods and to select from varied sources. She shares this lack of insight with many. However, if there has to be a food fixation, fish is a good choice. Dr. Snead describes it this way:

> Cereal depends on the quality of soil for its trace elements. But food from the sea, where there is an even mix, provides an excellent protein substance with natural protective additives. Iodine, for example, helps detoxify toxins found in fish. All seafood contains high amounts of mercury, some of it naturally. Fish preserved in the Smithsonian have the same percent of mercury as fish currently pulled from the sea. Fish have large amounts of

sulfur, a natural protector against mercury, and large amounts of zinc, which protect against cadmium. Everything in nature is a balance, and seafood is a perfect example of this.[32]

Family #3—The Harrises

SUMMARY

The Harris family has made many changes: They are involved in healthful food purchases, despite the fact that Dad is having problems adjusting to the new regime. Debbie and Danielle, the mischievous twins, try to get their parents to buy recently banned items.

GOOD BEHAVIOR'S REWARD

We have all been rewarded with food for good behavior. Many of us reward ourselves. Positive food enforcement is practiced by most cultures. Perhaps humanity will never understand why we do this. But if we must use food in this manner, we should at least use the *right* foods. And so the Harrises are attempting to reprogram their family.

PETER HARRIS' INNER CRY

When Peter Harris reveals his secret desire for the "bad" foods, it is not much different than telling his children not to steal, and then stealing with the back hand. It's difficult to train children when parents haven't totally accepted the new concepts. After all, our whole culture is not in tempo with the importance of better eating habits. How can we expect full cooperation from the children when we embark on this extraordinary change of behavior if they see the lack of acceptance at home? The failure of the Harrises' efforts are demonstrated in the success of the children sneaking the doughnuts in spite of their parents' opposition. For the Harris family, we are back to square one, with the need for more education. But education will only help those who *want* to change. And again, we must recognize that total change occurs slowly.

Studies show that the women of the family are more likely to be open and sensitive to information about food as they attempt to meet the nutritional needs of the family. When husbands perceive their wives as having an influence on their eating practices, their diets are usually better than average.[33] Food habits will change rapidly when immediate benefits are demonstrated.[34] Therefore, do your homework: List the benefits. Use this fact to full advantage.

THE HOLIDAY'S REWARD

Foods prohibited on ordinary days become the holiday's reward. How do we alter the children's practices when we sanction the objectionable customs by accompanying them with pleasure: the pleasure of holidays, the pleasure of company, and even the pleasure of going to the movies (popcorn, etc.)? Why must we regress when we celebrate?

As for entertaining, you would probably be more than happy to have good food for your guests, but would feel uncomfortable when friends come to your home expecting foods that are not available, such as coffee at the end of the meal. Chances are that if you did not plan a sweet dessert, someone would bring a cake anyway. Can you insult your visitors by not serving it? What is the solution?

One possibility is to go "all out." Prepare very special, but wholesome platters. The food presentations can be so magnificent in taste and appearance—no one would guess they are also highly nutritious. This is not to say that you want to fool people. On the contrary, you especially want your guests to know that healthful food can also be delicious. But what is more important is that you want your *children* to feel good about good food. Don't hide the fact that the food is, in fact, of superior nutritional quality. Your children will get the message if you are "up front" about it. We do not believe that healthful ingredients should be "sneaked" into meal plans.

For your own private family celebrations, you can make up holiday rituals that are filled with fun and express love without dependence on junk food. Preparing good foods in festive fashion takes added effort—but only until you learn a few tricks. A positive atmosphere with beautiful, nutrient-giving foods will earmark good eating habits with the pleasure of the occasion. If you never bake bread during the year, bake a natural bread for the holidays. A home-baked bread, offered as the highest reward (rather than the chocolate cake as the grand prize of the meal), will fill the house with superb smells, and with delighted exclamations from all. Trust us—this will really happen! Children will construe the bread as a premium, and associate it with pleasurable memories. You are now coupling emotional prizes (pleasure and fun) with *good food.*

THE SACRIFICE

Years ago a child might have bartered a dose of cod-liver oil for permission to visit a friend. The Harris twins see the *salad* as the sacrifice. Salad is no longer a food to be eaten because it is good or enjoyable. It is a concession for the parents' acceptance of junk food.

DEBBIE AND DANIELLE AND BEHAVIOR

Much of the girls' clowning could have been avoided if they were involved in decision-making at the supermarket. Using their ideas, they could be asked to participate. Children have come up with suggestions such as:

1) Selecting the whole-grain bread—finding the one with the least amount of additives. (Since breads are loaded with additives, this chore could occupy the twins right up to checkout time.)
2) If money is an issue, selecting the most healthful bread within a specific price range.
3) Gathering the fruits and vegetables on the shopping list. (This will keep them away from the danger areas for awhile.)
4) For older children, researching the unit cost of various brands of paper products; selecting the best buys.
5) Reading labels for all purchases.

Children should not feel as though they are being dragged along on the shopping excursion. Allow enough time to enable them to be part of the process. Children are more willing to eat foods if they have helped in their preparation. Let them wash, chop, mix, and pour. It will take patience and time, but how else are we going to battle the forces pulling in the other direction?

You can set standards for good food habits and still give the children the feeling that they are being respected, and that you are listening to them. The food disciplines do not have to be out of context with the listening and caring.

Family # 4—The Garcias

SUMMARY

Helen admits previous errors in food selection. Son Paul requests white bread sandwiches so he'll be "one of the guys." Helen agrees, and is later pleased at Paul's interest in healthful eating. Daughter Lisa selects a ready-mix for her birthday cake.

HELEN'S MEMORIES

Lisa is challenging her mother because she used to buy foods that they now know are unhealthful. Helen has been learning the concepts of better nutrition for several years. She fully appreciates their importance for the well-being of her children. She interprets her daughter's comments as criticism. By admitting the error of her ways, Helen anticipates gaining the respect of her children.

However, Helen missed the point that Lisa was also expressing her feelings about not getting the preferred junk foods anymore. Helen's response could have been improved by adding a reflective comment, such as, "You wish you could have foods you had when you were younger, don't you?" This is an example of an opportunity for you to be entirely true to *your* own feelings, and at the same time respect and understand your *child's* reactions. It should be a comfort to you that you are not alone. You are not a "bad" parent if you cannot bring about the food change in one stride. Children will resist and complain—even years later. Allow them to express their feelings. Recognize and accept such expression—it's bound to happen.

PAUL'S SANDWICH

Paul has requested white bread for his sandwiches. Helen has decided that the stress of Paul's anticipation of peer pressure is more important than the stress of eating nutrient-deficient white bread. As a parent, only you can be the judge in an either-or situation. You alone can gauge whether or not a particular indiscretion will throw the nutritional scale off balance. When you are having trouble with a decision, let your children know about it. Instead of saying, "I know what's right," you could say, "It's hard for me to decide. I know what I want and I know what you want, so we'll compromise today." Stating your feelings about the trade-off can be very helpful.

It's nice that Paul is able to communicate so openly with his mother. His ability to do this suggests that he probably won't have to make concessions too much longer. He will have the strength and confidence to face his friends with his own values at an earlier age than most teenagers. Helen is wise to recognize the fact that individuality is not a quality of young people. It is an attribute of adults, and takes time to develop. People who want to break away from a detrimental pattern need courage. Children do not necessarily have that courage.

We know one mother who handled a similar situation another way. Her daughter was the object of derision from classmates because her lunches were so different. (At any rate, that's what the child reported. There was a lot of competition among these girls, so it's hard to ascertain what the real motivations were.) Her mother encouraged her to develop an attitude of amusement. Instead of being upset, this child picked up her friends' packages of Twinkies, ding-dongs, or whatever, and read the labels to the other classmates. Her friends began to question their own lunchboxes. Although turning tables happened to work in this case, there are dangers inherent in such an approach. A child may not feel as though he or she is being taken seriously when parents treat the dilemma with humor. When children are stressed, they don't want their feelings sloughed off with merriment. In addition, this maneuver is similar to telling your child to hit back, and using force is no way to solve problems.

When our own son was thirteen, he made a similar request concerning the bread used for sandwiches. However, since he was thoroughly integrated in the world of good nutrition since birth (with older siblings as his support system), Michael requested that we use one slice of white bread, and one slice of whole-wheat bread for his sandwiches. "If I eat the sandwich *white side out,* no one will notice." Michael did not want to miss out on his nutrients, but figured quite literally that half a loaf is better than none. But then Michael always displayed a practical nature. One rainy day he could only find one of his boots. He wore the one boot, saying, "Why should both feet get wet?"

PAUL'S TRANSITIONS

Dr. Serafina Corsello comments on Paul's transitions:

> There is no doubt that when you remove something that is dear to a child (and junk food is indeed dear to the hearts of children), you are removing an important love object. The difficulty is accentuated because of the acceptance of junk foods by the media, by peers, and by most American homes.
>
> You might even liken its removal to that of killing a pet. Therefore, you have to be cognizant of the fact that the child will go through stages of adaptation. It is beautiful to see how Paul went through a period of rebellion and denial to probable depression, to his current endorsement of nutrition. His acceptance is accompanied by a little bargaining. Eventually he will reach total subscription to the nutrition-good-health concept. You can see it happening already.
>
> Paul will accept the loss of the love object (the junk food), and it will be the love object of his childhood—the eating habits of a child. He will be able to internalize an error of an age passed, an age gone by. And he will be able to do so because his parents have accepted their own mistakes. He will reach levels of greater awareness as he continues to be educated—as he continues to learn the importance of nutrition and the validity of proper concepts of healthful eating. Paul promises to be a new link to good ecological internal cleansing. This is a good success story.[35]

LISA'S BIRTHDAY CAKE

Lisa's request for a candy bar was an effort to test limits. As Helen thought about what happened, she knew she could have clarified her values more precisely. The Garcias are far enough along in the food transition to establish ground rules that should be different from those set by the novice Smithers family.

Limits for your child's birthday party should be no different from those set for other special family occasions. You can promote a great deal of confusion if you impart this message: On 364 days of the year, you eat excellent food, but on your birthday you may eat garbage. Instead, *the food should reflect the specialness of the event.*

Celebrations, however, are so often out of the house—they're someone else's birthday party. You don't want to say, "You have to go to the party and be different." But you can negotiate, and expect a price: You can carefully manage the diet before and after (more salads, more raw foods, etc.). Feed the children before they leave. With stomachs full of good food, there's less room for junk. Dr. Lendon Smith prescribes the following as a before-party regimen:

> Serve your children peanuts, meat, fish or eggs. These are long-term energy sources. Give them 500 milligrams of vitamin C, some B_6, or the whole B-complex; about 500 milligrams of calcium. They will not be as quick to jump into the sweet stuff and overeat.

In spite of all your precautions, don't be disappointed if your children still "pig out." Don't expect more restraint than they can handle—don't expect what is unreasonable. A certain amount of humility is necessary on your part. Don't anticipate perfection from your children in this kind of party situation. A healthy child will probably dig into the junk food, at least to some extent. It's so easy to become arrogant and self-righteous when you've discovered the true way. *Now* is the time to maintain a sense of humor and a sense of proportion. With the exception of emergencies, it is far better to invite discussions than to give commands, and to know when to get out of the way.

At this point, the best friend you have is *nature*. Many parents report that an interesting phenomenon begins to occur when children are on toxin-free diets. They become acutely sensitive to the junk foods when they do indulge. They suffer headaches, stomachaches, and general feelings of malaise. It is not hard to associate the ill feelings with the party food. As they get older, they begin to curtail their intake of these foods. It's a natural process. (By the way, this does not mean that junk food eaters are less sensitive. They have simply *maladapted*, and are not as keenly aware of body chemistry changes.)

PAUL'S COMPLEXION

Children's vanity can be used to advantage, especially as they get a little older. Good nutrition means good posture. It means clear complexion. It means beautiful hair. It means better vision. It means brighter eyes. It means being thinner.

Our own children noticed that when teenage friends' acne was widespread, *they* had peaches-and-cream complexions. When one of our sons went to Europe at age 16 with the school chorus, he was the *last* to get sick, and his illness was mild. Everyone else suffered severely. These manifestations of good-food regimens will do more to reinforce the facts than any words of wisdom.

Paul appears to be further along in his transitions than his sister. It may be because he is older, but individual differences should not be overlooked. Lisa may have more allergies, and possibly more cravings. The experiences she has with her friends or teachers may be different from those of her brother. The lesson here is to avoid comparisons. What may be easy for Paul could be very difficult for Lisa.

Family #5—The Davises

SUMMARY

Tom, pushing Linda and the groceries in the supermarket wagon, meets a neighbor who is chasing after his "terrible twos" daughter. Tom expounds on the media "booby trap." Linda, only a year-and-a-half old, displays the media influence when she sings one of the commercial cereal jingles, heard on TV.

SIBLING RIVALRY

Dr. Corsello comments on the encounter between Tom and his neighbor:

> This is the story of young fathers who have become more aware of food content. The men are talking "childrenese." The conversation centers around the supermarket behavior of their daughters. It is fascinating to see how Tom counsels his friend. They discuss coping with the development of children's eating habits, and even regression, which has focused around food (the result of the threat of a new sibling).
> Sibling rivalry often expresses itself in the aggressive drive, the older child punching the little one. (I personally tried to poke my brother's eyes out. I didn't grab food—I grabbed his eyes. This was more direct. I wasn't going to punish myself, I was going to punish the baby.) Linda, Tom's older daughter, had her parents perfectly pegged. She went into regressive eating habits, knowing that she would hurt them that way. The Cain and Abel story of

sibling rivalry is the story of all human beings. At age three Linda was so aware of nutrition that she could say, "That's yukky," or "Preservatives." At that young age she had learned that certain foods were very damaging. In her regression, she reaches for anything that is bad for her, and does so with much glory. (One wants to know what will happen once she gets over the sibling rivalry.)

BECKY

Dr. Corsello discusses Becky, the neighbor's child:

Becky is going through the terrible twos' stage. With the junk food on the lower shelves, Gerry is trying to curtail her grabbing habits. And he thinks that Tom has had it so easy! Tom gives his friend a little course in child development and in shopping expectations. The most important message that Tom offers is that children, try as you will to steer them away from junk food, are influenced by the media "booby trap." The young children are in the precognizant stage of awareness. The booby trap has so brainwashed the little angels that the parents have little power or control, unless they keep the child away from both the TV and the junk food.

Reinforcing Dr. Corsello's observations is the fact that young children are largely prisoners of visual input. They accept what they see without the ability to judge, or to relate cause and effect. They cannot separate the commercial message from the story content. (Again, we suggest studying Piaget, who offers insight into the development of intelligence, helping you understand the qualitative differences at various stages of growth. See Appendix.)[36] The flame is fanned when junk food is associated with music, strengthening the power of suggestion. Madison Avenue is well versed in this aspect of advertising. Tom feels totally helpless when faced with his child's ability to recognize the cereal tune and sing it out—a feeling he has already imparted to his neighbor.

THE GRANDPARENTS

We all know that grandparents have difficulty saying "No" to their grandchildren. Dr. Corsello explains the grandparent-grandchild phenomenon:

Grandparents by nature love to give in, especially when the grandchildren give them "the eyes" and say "please." Children know how to manipulate grandparents. The children are being brainwashed with the "goodness" of the junk food, and this is exactly what they obtain from the grandparents.

You don't want to deprive your children of the special grandparent relationship. This is one of the best facets of a loving support system any child can have. But there can be real battles between parents and grandparents, and the child is the pawn. You can explain to the loving, adoring grandparents that they can buy nuts, or some types of cookies (carob, oatmeal, certain brands of peanut butter cookies), so that they can actually indulge in their hobby (catering to the grandchildren), but they can do so with foods that are not damaging. And here again we see the importance of collective education—education for the entire culture.

As a child, my whims were favored by my grandmother. However, some cultures are more in tune with natural foods: I was given carob pods to chew, which satisfied my oral needs and my sweet tooth, and my grandmother's desire to please me.

In the American culture (and a few European cultures as well), the grandparent-child relationship has a special quality because the grandparents are in the same stage of development as the children. The children are on their way up to maturity, heading toward adult integration. The grandparents are on their way down from responsibility. They meet each other on the same level. The grandparents have transferred their obligations to their children, which allows them time to be more indulging. Coming away from family duties, they meet with the grandchildren at the same polarity of self-actual needs.

Grandparents are usually at a stage where they are watching their diets. How convenient to transfer this need to that little something they love, who, in fact (in the grandparents' view) needs to gain body weight and strength and height. This justifies the giving of food! It's a natural, spontaneous game of the evolution of human behavior. If you, as parent, are caught in the middle, attempt to make *your* parents aware that the children need *better* food. You then shift the *quality,* not the *emphasis.* The game, of course, is played forever. Just as grandparents on the floor are really playing for themselves (not the child), they are feeding the child for themselves.

TELEVISION AND MAVERICKS

Dr. Corsello concludes her comments with a general discussion of TV and of families who oppose the mainstream of culture:

When most of the children knew all about every TV program, my daughter had only a limited exposure. This deprived her of social contact of a commonality. It is very difficult to be a purist in a culture that is so far away from your views. You must constantly touch base with the mainstream of the culture. The child should be made aware that the mainstream might not be optimal. But at the same time, you have to recognize that your child will not trust you entirely. You are only one person (or two), and the mainstream of culture is the herd.

Anyone who departs from the herd, even among animals, will have difficulties. As much as the child loves the mother and/or father, the security is still in the herd. And the herd (the old peer influence with adolescence) may be moving away from the *family* herd. Children attempt to create new herds of their own. They do this by testing their ability to satellite out of the main family herd. They now form little herds with their peers. Their values become the values of the peers. They collide completely with the primary herd of the family. Then you have a battle—a tremendous conflict. Where does this leave nutrition if the family is engaged in completely pure, one hundred percent adherence—and the herd is totally unempathic and removed from the concept? Who is the child going to believe? Do you think the child will go back to the family and never dare get out into the satellite to form new herds and new nuclear families? Or will the child reject the family and join the peers? And this is only *one* area of conflict—only one area of our endeavor: nutrition!

Dr. Corsello's caveats and messages are well taken. The support group is lacking. There is no cultural backup. We must acknowledge the problem and concentrate on how to cope with it. We have to develop systems for living with it. The family can withstand this if it is close-knit. Children will interject their parents' values when the family unit is tight and strong. The more clarity on the part of the parents in stating and *living* their beliefs, the more potential for the children sharing those beliefs. A critical aspect of growing up is for children to examine their parents' values, possibly to rebel against them, and then to reestablish their own values. Through respect, love, attention, and nurturing, parents foster strength in children. Children with strong egos will be able to use outside influences (including those from peers) better than children who feel shaky about themselves.

MORE ON TELEVISION

Because television plays such a powerful role, it is important for everyone to understand its total soul and sovereignty. The following statements from educators, and from those who appeared at the Council on Children, Media and Merchandising for the Select Committee on Nutrition and Human Needs of the United States Senate, should be helpful:

☆ Michael Kamen (our education consultant) advises that because children get strong messages from television, it is important for them to understand the media: Talk about the conflicts. Let your children know that commercials are produced by people who want to make money.

Aside from the content, the very act of watching television is detrimental. It is a passive activity that does not require interaction with the environment. This means the child is not responsible for having control of his or her activities. The specially designed colorful action is in conflict with learning how to relate to the real world. One solution? Don't have a television set when children are part of your family structure. Does that sound unreasonable? At the very least, TV should not be available to *young* children. For further reference, read *Four Arguments for the Elimination of Television* by Jerry Mander, Morrow-Quill Paperbacks, New York, 1978.

☆ Advertisers spend over $600 million a year selling to children on television.[37]

☆ Over a million young children are still watching television at midnight.[38]

☆ Over half of the TV ads directed to children are for highly sugared foods, but none of these ads tell children that sugar can cause cavities.[39]

☆ TV ranks as the most powerful selling medium in America. The food industry dominates this medium. One out of five commercials advertises food or beverage products. . . . To children, TV ads promise fun and excitement, an "adventure in every bite."[40]

☆ The average preschooler watches just under 30 hours of TV a week. Even if it was terrific TV, that's entirely too much. . . . Children can't make fine-line distinctions—advertising for them is uniquely deceptive.[41]

☆ The more television viewing children do, the more likely they are to eat heavily sugared cereals, and the more often they eat between meals. They also consume more total snack foods, and eat more candy and chips and other empty-calorie foods.[42]

☆ Children will respond to and remember fragments of information that are often repeated, spoken by real or animated authority figures, or that seem to satisfy an impulsive need. The latter may be an explanation for children's fascination and recall of food commercials.[43]

☆ Those children who watch more commercial television at home request more items at the supermarket. The fact that the food product most frequently requested by the children, namely cereals, corresponds to the food product most frequently advertised in commercials directed at children provides additional support for the hypothesis of a causal relationship between television ads and children's food requests and preferences.[44] (However, don't overlook the fact that, although television has its impact, the greatest influence is your example. Most of children's eating habits are learned from adult behavior.)

☆ The relationship of voice to visual on a mix, that is, sound effect mix to visual, is a major factor in determining the way in which the material will be approached by the viewer. As an illustration, if you were to play bright joyful dance music in the murder scene in *Psycho*, the terror component of the action would be substantially less than the sound effect that was created therein.[45]

These statements demonstrate that fighting the subliminal imprinting of the powerful selling maneuvers with both visual and auditory messages is no easy task. Action for Children's Television in Boston offers this advice:

> Don't just turn on television. Turn on a program, and turn off the set when the program is over. Help your children choose the programs they watch, and watch with them when you can. Use the programs you and your children watch as a jumping-off point for family discussions. Set a limit on the amount of TV your children watch. When you are at work or out in the evenings, tell the babysitter how to handle TV viewing. Check the schedule on your public TV station for creative noncommercial alternatives. When you don't like what TV is teaching, turn it off. Remember, *you control the set*.[46]

We know that many parents today are rushed, and some of the suggestions may seem impossible. You may not have the support systems your parents had. If you do not have the time or the patience or the inclination to engage in the kind of communication that has been outlined, it is best to shop alone. If you feel pressured at the end of the workday, and that is when you have to shop, make arrangements for your children, and do your marketing without them. Although not ideal, this is better than fighting, better than screaming, better than having to give in to the purchase of the junk foods.

It is unfair to scream at a child who is being brainwashed by such powerful authorities. And be aware that when environmental factors have a lesser role, TV plays a greater role. Dr. Reis agrees that children who make demands in the supermarket, or make the shopping excursion more difficult, should indeed remain at home. He says:

> Part of growing up is learning to be frustrated. Everyone wants more than he or she has (including the parents who desire the Mercedes, a better job, a raise, a better sex life, etc.), and children need to learn that they are not going to get everything they want. Instead of being tyrannized, you the parent should establish a range of free choices, and let your child make decisions within that range. Example: if there are 4 or 5 cereal varieties that are acceptable to you, let your child select from the list. If none of the choices are satisfactory to the children, you will have to deal with resentment. When you limit your children's world, they may have to conform, but they should not be required to like it.[47]

Family #6—The Barrons

SUMMARY

Irene Barron is a single parent on a tight budget. She meets neighbors who are "coupon shopping." Her daughter Susie wishes Mom could buy some pretty soap instead of the large cakes that are not as exciting but are economical.

WATCHING THE BUDGET

If Irene Barron could read the recipe section of this book, she would know she could shop for nutritious foods that are inexpensive and easy to prepare. It is sad that grain and bean dishes are considered low-status foods in our country. Bean and grain dishes can be varied, nutrient-giving, filling, and delicious. Furthermore, *they stretch the dollar.*

Irene might even have money left over to treat Susie to the pretty soap.

As for the coupon ladies, they should learn that *food that doesn't nourish you is never a bargain.* For the average American family, there is little association between socioeconomic status and the nutritional quality of the diet.[48] The difference is not in your pocketbook, but rather on your focus. Those who consider their food selections based on *cost* consume more calories. The overall quality of these diets is lower.[49] Those who consider *nutrition* have improved diets, and may or may not spend more. For those on a budget, the preparation of a list is the best tool. This eliminates impulse buying.

IRENE'S CONVENIENCE FOOD

Irene's purchase of frozen TV dinners reminds us of our children's pet tease: They tell everyone that nostalgia for them is "frozen in the middle." (We have long since unplugged the freezer.) Another incident occurred years back when our neighbor, seven years old, came to tell us she had hurt her fingers while helping her mother prepare dinner. "Oh, did you burn yourself?" we asked. "No," she replied, "My fingers got frostbitten."

Of course frozen foods are a convenience for busy parents. But again there are no signs in the supermarket indicating the nutrient losses caused by the freezing process. The subtle message inherent in the difference in the prices of fresh foods versus frozen is that you are paying for packaging and high technology. (See Table 7.) Grains and beans and seeds are *natural* convenience foods. They can be stored for long periods of time. Harvest is only once a year.

Family #7—The Chapmans

SUMMARY

Beth, a pure nutrition advocate, meets a "soulmate" in the supermarket.

Beth avoids conflict by being a "closet" nutrition advocate because of the stigma attached to being so different. Until the importance of nu-

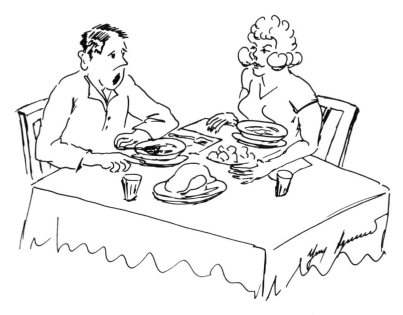

This is delicious. Did you defrost it yourself?

trition education becomes paramount in the entire culture, people like Beth go about their business doing what they have to do, often keeping their lifestyles top-secret. However, if you are envisioning a nation full of clandestine "Beths" furtively rushing about in hush-hush fashion, fear not. Very few people are well informed about nutrition, and many are misinformed.

Dr. R. Lehmann of Columbia University reveals interesting information in a study entitled "Nutritional Knowledge, Attitudes and Food Consumption Patterns of U.S. Female Heads of Households." He shows that personal experience is by far the most important source of nutritional information. Learning from labels on packages runs a close second.[50]

It's unfortunate that many foods are "Standards." Standard products do not require ingredient listings. There are many food industry ploys used to avoid accurate labeling, such as secondary additives, "cover" names that imply that the additive is something different, etc. For Beth and her friend, the problem is not so much finding healthful food, but finding convincing ways to pass the word on to other parents.

Twenty-four hundred years ago Euripides said:

I think that fortune watches over our lives, Surer than we.
But well said: he who strives will find his gods strive for him equally.

Chapter 3

CHOICES IN THE SUPERMARKET

Many a dangerous temptation comes to us in fine gay colors that are but skin-deep.
—*Commentaries*, Genesis, III

The White Tornado, Mr. Clean, Mrs. Butterworth, Aunt Jemima, and Josephine the Plumber drop in on American kitchens. We decided to do the same and visit the Smithers in the role of Good Food Gurus. (If Madison Avenue was staging the visit, we would be dubbed something like Swami Tell-Me Howe and Maharishi Health-Wealth.)

The Smithers, you may remember, are Ellen and Bob, and their children: Judy (15), Robbie (13), Jennifer (10), John (8), and Sherry (5).

The Scenario

Kamens: Good morning to all the Smithers. There's an old joke about those who get up in the morning and say, "Good morning, Lord," and others who, upon rising, say, "Good Lord, morning!" Sometimes the difference between a happy or unhappy outlook when facing the day may be directly related to what you eat.
Sherry: What you *eat?*
Robbie: That means Judy eats all the wrong things.
Judy: Look who's talking. You're the prize crab.
Mom: Children, please. Don't make me feel like my neighbor. Some one said to her, "If you had it to do over again, would you have chil-

dren?" She answered, "Yes, but not the same ones." Are there any foods which prevent siblings from taunting each other?

Kamens: We're accustomed to teasing. We have a large family too. Let's talk about your first food choices of the day: What you have for breakfast.

Judy: I don't have any breakfast.

Kamens: You and too many others start the day without breakfast. Would you expect your Mom or Dad to drive the car on an empty gas tank? That's exactly what you are doing when you go without breakfast, or when you have a poor breakfast.

Judy: The car won't start without gas, but I can move around without breakfast.

Kamens: But *how* do you move? How clearly do you *think?* How well do you perform? With a good breakfast, you have more energy for a longer time. A study was done on typists to determine the effects of breakfast on their performance. One group of typists had no breakfast; the other had a highly nutritious breakfast. There was no question about the superiority of the breakfast eaters. They made fewer mistakes and were much faster. They retained this advantage until mid-afternoon.

Statistics also show you will have better *long-range* health if you eat a wholesome breakfast every day. So whatever it is you do—play baseball or tennis, go jogging, do housework, read, dance—you'll do it better if you start the day with high-test fuel: a good breakfast.

John: You mean I'll get better grades if I have a really good breakfast?[1, 2]

Kamens: Does that sound surprising? It may be true!

John: What if I have a breakfast bar? That's an easy breakfast, but Mom won't let me eat that kind of food.

Kamens: John, *what* you eat is important. A number of years ago a study conducted in Iowa proved that children who have a *good* breakfast (one that includes protein) actually perform better than those who don't eat as well.[3] A very popular breakfast bar is nothing more than fortified candy. Eighty percent of its calories come from fat and sugar. This type of breakfast is totally lacking in the necessary amount of protein, fiber and nutrients that help you function better.[4]

Judy, some people need a little more time to move around before they have an appetite at the start of the day. Find some chores to do before you reach the kitchen. This may help get your appetite going. There are also trick recipes for people like you, Judy—recipes for preparing light, easy-down foods. (See the recipe section under "breakfast ideas for the non-breakfast eater.")

Judy: So come on, Mom. We'll all be scholars if you make us bacon and eggs every day, and fresh-squeezed orange juice.

Robbie: And toast and pancakes.

Jennifer: And milkshakes.

Sherry: I might even get to be the first lady President.

John: Or an astronaut.

Kamens: You children have outlined a breakfast full of protein, fat, and carbohydrate. You even included fiber, but within the realm of all that good food, there are still many choices to make. Let's start with your morning juice. If you choose commercially prepared orange juice, the kind that comes in frozen cans, containers or bottles, it might surprise you to learn that your glass of juice often contains almost no vitamin C. Vitamin C is a very fragile, unstable nutrient, which disappears quickly upon exposure to air, light, heat, and storage time.[5] In fact, vitamin C is so fragile, that if you cut an orange in half and leave it at room temperature for one half hour, 7 percent of its vitamin C will disappear.[6]

Mom: Are you saying we shouldn't have orange juice?

Kamens: Remember, we are talking about choices. Even if you

TABLE 17
BAR NONE

Ingredients of Popular Breakfast Bar

Ingredients: Sugar, partially hydrogenated vegetable oil (may contain one or more of the following oils: cottonseed, soybean, palm), dried corn syrup, invert sugar, peanut butter (peanuts, dextrose, vegetable monoglycerides, and salt), calcium caseinate, chocolate, peanuts, soy protein isolate, flour, glycerin, cocoa, nonfat milk, sodium ascorbate, magnesium hydroxide, salt, lecithin, artificial flavors, sodium stearoyl-2-lactylate, polysorbate 60, sorbitan monostearate, vitamin E, ferrous fumarate, vitamin A palmitate, niacinamide, zinc oxide, copper glucomate, preservatives (TBHG and citric acid), calcium pantothenate, thiamine mononitrate, vitamin B_{12}, pyrodoxine hydrochloride, folic acid.

squeeze the juice yourself, a whole orange is a better choice. There are two nutrition "laws of choice" that serve as guidelines. When you understand these rules, you will be able to answer many of your own questions about the quality of food.

Law of Choice # 1:   The more processed a food is, the fewer nutrients that food contains. (Select the least processed food.)

Law of Choice # 2:   Some foods should be avoided because they contain harmful ingredients. (Select the food with the least amount of harmful ingredients.)

There are a few amendments. For example, grains need to be cooked. (Yes, cooking is processing.) But these two laws, for the most part, are immutable.

Dad: In other words, some foods have additives, or unnatural substances, and other foods are lacking in vitamins and minerals. We should be aware of these two facts when we make our food choices.

Kamens: Exactly! Now back to the orange juice. Frozen juice is concentrated, which usually involves a four-step condensing procedure (oranges squeezed; water removed; the concentrate shipped; the water added for bottling in the state in which it is to be sold). Furthermore, the pulp is removed from most *frozen* juices, and orange juice in *containers* is pasteurized—heated at 190°F. It too may be condensed. We're talking about *many* processing steps. Bottled juice is pasteurized, cooled, and clarified through filters.[7, 8] This procedure gives the juice a shelf life of several months.

Sherry: You mean I drink *old* juice?

Robbie: Look, this container says "PASTEURIZED."

Mom: I never noticed that before.

Kamens: Advertising has convinced everyone that it is un-American to start the day without a glass of orange juice—regardless of where you live! The people of Montana are convinced that they must have oranges, even though they live long distances from orange groves. If fruits and vegetables are going to travel, they must be picked before they are ripe. This prevents them from spoiling on their pilgrimage to faraway states. However, when a fruit or vegetable is picked before it is fully ripe, there are nutrient losses.[9]

TABLE 18
NOW YOU "C" IT: NOW YOU DON'T

Specific Losses of Vitamin C Due to Temperature Treatment
Heating to 80° .... 23% loss
Initial freezing process .... 32% loss

Additional Causes of Vitamin C Losses

1) Temperature variations (cause of largest losses)
2) Food processing additives:
    Salt
    Sugar
    Enzymes
    Metal Catalysts
    Oxidants
    Amino Acids

From Robert S. Harris, and Endel Karmas, eds., *Nutritional Evaluation of Food Processing*, second edition (Westport, CT: The AVI Publishing Co., Inc., 1977), pp. 231, 267, and Owen R. Fennema, ed., *Principles of Food Sciences*, Part 1; Food Chemistry (New York: Marcel Dekker, Inc., 1976), pp. 361–66.

Dad: Does that mean no oranges unless we live in Florida or California?

Kamens: We are talking about choices, remember?

Dad: Ah, yes, Law #1. Eat the whole orange because it has more nutrients. But what about law #2—sprays, dyes, etc?

Kamens: Your best choice is still the whole orange. Bioflavonoids are a very important part of the C-complex vitamins, and they're found in the pulp of the orange. Eating the whole orange also provides fiber. It would be nice to eat oranges picked at peak—oranges that did not visit the beauty parlor.

Sherry:
John: THE BEAUTY PARLOR????
Jennifer:

Kamens: Green oranges are often dyed orange, and many oranges are coated with mineral oil or carnauba wax.[10] But you have to select from what is available, depending on where you live. The advantage of a whole orange is that its natural architectural form has not been altered. You consume it as nature intended.

John: When do we talk about eggs? I love eggs.

Kamens: Okay, let's talk about eggs! Recalling Law of Choice #1, how do you think eggs should be prepared?

Dad: The answer to a question is: Beginning to ask the right questions.

Robbie: Well, if cooking is considered processing, and processing takes away nutrition, should we eat *raw* eggs?

Sherry: I don't know if I can do that. The idea makes me queasy.

Kamens: From the standpoint of *nutrients,* raw eggs would be your best choice.[11] Your great grandfather probably drank raw eggs right from the shell, Sherry, and your great grandmother may have cracked them into drinks. In fact, many people still use raw eggs in special beverage mixes.

Some nutrition specialists are concerned about a substance in raw eggs called avidin. Avidin destroys an imporant nutrient called biotin. There is a controversy as to whether or not the egg should be heated in boiling water for 20 seconds to reduce the avidin. Dr. Richard Wurtman, professor of endocrinology at M.I.T., says: "Production of biotin deficiency in (humans) requires the use of egg white in quantities supplying as much as 30 percent of the energy requirement and most of the dietary protein."[12] So it doesn't appear to be much of a problem, unless you are consuming tremendous quantities of raw eggs. Many people heat eggs for a short time in hopes of eliminating the risk of food poisoning from contamination, which occurs when sanitation standards are not up to par at chicken farms.[13]

Dr. C. T. Smith of the American College of Applied Clinical Nutriton, reports that raw eggs are not as easily digested as cooked eggs. He says: "When we cook the white of an egg, the protein is handled more easily by the digestive system. The cooking also destroys parasites which hinder the absorption of nutrients. However, cooking destroys beneficial enzymes along with harmful enzymes."[14]

So you see it's a trade-off. You give and you get. That's why your diet should consist of both raw and lightly cooked foods.

Sherry: I'm *not* eating raw eggs!

Kamens: We appreciate your feelings. Let's remember the law, though. If your egg is cooked so that the yolk is still soft, the egg will

have more nutrients.[15] That means your eggs could be lightly steamed, poached or "looking at you."
Robbie: What about hard-boiled eggs?
Kamens: A hard-cooked egg is not as beneficial as an egg prepared with a runny yolk. But it is still an excellent food. By the way, if you do use hard-cooked eggs, *steam* them to hardness. Don't boil them. The yolk will be mellower.

Technology is responsible for major changes from the traditional forms of food nourishment, as was shown by the results of an interesting study from the University of Illinois. Headed by Dr. Fred Kummerow, the researchers observed the differences in test animals when they were fed farm-fresh eggs and an egg substitute.[16] The difference in the rats was striking. The rats fed the egg substitute were smaller, distorted, and showed stunted growth, plus hair loss, diarrhea and premature death.

Food chemists are able to tell us exactly what chemicals foods are made of, but they cannot take these chemicals and manufacture a real apple, a real orange, or *a real egg*. Egg substitute is a product that looks and tastes like scrambled eggs, and is promoted as "healthful." *Caveat emptor.* (Let the buyer beware.)
Robbie: Were the rats on the egg substitute fed anything else? What I'm asking is this: Would I eat as much of such a product as the rats ate?
Kamens: A good question, Robbie. Even if the rats were fed nothing else, the experiment is still valid and important. It points to the difference in the results between feeding the animals whole real food (the farm-fresh eggs) and the nonfood diet (the chemicalized product). Since similar changes are being made in much of the processed food you are eating, it is possible for all your meals to be fabricated. You could go through a lifetime eating only this kind of food—ersatz food, lacking in good, true nutrition.[17] We just don't have the ability to handle these alien molecules. It's like trying to run a car on soda pop.
Dad: You didn't say anything about cholesterol. How many eggs could we eat with safety?
Kamens: Blaming eggs as a cause of heart disease is no longer as popular a theory as it once was. More and more evidence demonstrates that it's the refined, sugar-laden, overprocessed foods that may be responsible for dangerous cholesterol levels.

Dad: You're kidding! You mean I've been cutting back on eggs for no reason?

Kamens: Since the issue has become so confused, let's call for some help. We'll go to prestigious researchers and doctors.

☆ American Medical Association: "The anti-fat, anti-cholesterol fad is not just foolish and futile. . . . It also carries some risk."[18]

☆ *New England Journal of Medicine,* Dr. George V. Mann: "Trials have failed to show more than a trivial effect of diet on cholesterolemia [high cholesterol levels]."[19]

☆ Massachusetts Institute of Technology, Neurophysiologists Edward R. Gruberg and Dr. Stephen A. Raymond: "Cholesterol is universally present in . . . all animal cells. All human cells can make cholesterol. Diet accounts for a relatively small fraction of the total amount of cholesterol in the body."[20]

☆ The Himalayan International Institute, Dr. Rudolph Ballentine: "Egg yolks not only contain cholesterol in significant quantities, they also contain lecithin. Lecithin is an unusual fat-like compound which has the special property of being able to dissolve cholesterol and other fats."[21]

☆ *Journal of the American Medical Association,* Dr. Allen Nichols: "It is not true that coronary heart disease decreases on a cholesterol-lowering diet."[22]

☆ *American Journal of Clinical Nutrition,* Dr. J. Hautvast: "In most individuals the egg is of small importance in elevating blood cholesterol."[23]

☆ Archives of Pathological Laboratory Medicine, Drs. Kamio and Kummerow: "The aorta (the main blood vessel) from humans subjected to elective coronary bypass surgery exhibited the same type of pathology as [test animals] that had never been fed cholesterol or saturated fat."[24]

☆ University of Illinois, Dr. Fred Kummerow: ". . . Cholesterol [is] so essential to life that it is [manufactured in the body] to assure adequate levels of tissue structure and function. . . . Cholesterol serves as a structural component and as a functional component in every cell in the body. It serves as a structural component in the skin and provides it the properties to shed water. It also insulates brain and nerve cells . . . so that stimuli can be carried from nerve endings for interpretation by the brain."[25]

☆ *American Journal of Clinical Nutrition*, Drs. Barbara O'Brien and Raymond Reiser: "Conscientious adherence to a low cholesterol fish and poultry diet failed to change blood cholesterol concentrations beyond the normal range of variability for the majority of those checked. In other words, dietary changes that eliminated a high cholesterol food (in this case meat) had no effect on the cholesterol levels."[26]

☆ *Lancet*, Dr. Jon A. Story and Dr. David Kritchevsky: "In the physiological complexities attendant on cholesterol metabolism, it is rare to see simple cause and effect results."[27] [This referred to consumption of eggs and rise in cholesterol.]

John: Oh boy! All the eggs we want!

Mom: It will certainly help my food budget.

Kamens: Eggs sell for about 65¢ a pound—you are getting a *high protein food.* Although we are talking *breakfast,* the egg can also be used for lunches, dinners, and even snacks. By the way, although we have shown that cholesterol in the diet does not relate to heart disease, it's of interest to note that fried and hard-cooked eggs produce higher blood cholesterol levels in test animals than eggs prepared other ways. When eggs are lightly scrambled or baked, they don't cause as high a rise in cholesterol as the fried or hard eggs. When the eggs are raw or soft-boiled, there is an almost insignificant increase.[28]

Jennifer: Law #1!

Mom: I always had a feeling that eggs would partially compensate for some of the junk foods the kids are exposed to.

Kamens: Your intuitive sense was correct. Dr. Jeffrey Bland, a well-known biochemist, sums it up by saying, "The quick removal of the egg from our diet may be an example of throwing out the baby with the bath water."[29]

Judy: This has nothing to do with eggs, but I confused "diet" with "nutrition" on a health class test. How would you define these words?

Sherry: I know, nutrition is vegetables.

John: No. Nutrition is anything that tastes yukky.

Jennifer: Nutrition means it's not candy.

Kamens: Diet is the food you eat. Nutrition is the study of what happens to food after you eat it: what the food does for you or what it does to you. I hope you will soon learn that good food—food that's nutritious—can also be delicious!

Robbie: So now that we've settled the egg issue, let's sizzle the bacon.

Kamens: Well . . . Bacon is a food that has fewer nutrients per serving than most other meats. It is mostly fat and it's laced with nitrites. It isn't exactly high-test fuel.[30]

Dad: Are nitrites harmful? I thought the experts changed their minds about them, and said they're not so bad after all.

Kamens: Nitrites can combine with natural stomach and food substances to cause powerful cancer-causing agents.[31] The F.D.A. considered banning nitrites in light of test results from an M.I.T. study showing that nitrite produces cancer of the lymphatic system.[32] But the F.D.A. reversed its decision to phase out the nitrites. Dr. Paul Newberne, the researcher who performed the studies, claims that the decision was reversed because of pressure from the powerful meat industry, which in turn claimed that it would suffer severe economic hardships as a consequence of nitrite phase-out. Yet other countries have banned the additive. In fact, some countries do not buy U.S. meat because of their nitrite content. As you know, nitrites are found in sausages, hot dogs, cold cuts, many other varieties of meat, and *bacon.*

Dad: Don't the nitrites prevent botulism?

Kamens: Yes. In addition to rendering a pretty pink color to meats, nitrites do have the effect of *preserving.* However, there are meat products on the market that do not contain nitrites, and they are safe. Good manufacturing practices eliminate any danger. The use of nitrites may encourage sloppy practices.

Judy: I learned in science that there are nitrites in foods naturally.

Kamens: There is no evidence of nitrite toxicity from vegetables. This may be because the presence of ascorbic acid in natural foods is protective.[33] Once again, we see the order and plan in natural foods and the price we pay when we tamper with their "wholeness." It is interesting to note that vitamin C prevents stomach cancer caused by the nitrites in various products, including pickled vegetables and dried, salted fish.[34] When foods are cooked, the nitrosamines (carcinogens caused by the nitrites) become even more concentrated.[35]

Robbie: My friend eats funny frankfurters. They're gray. He says they're healthier.

Kamens: Those are nitrite-free franks. They taste exactly the same as the red ones. You see, the nitrites are used basically for cosmetic purposes. Our children used to call nitrite-free franks "albino" frankfurters. Paul Newberne says that the nitrite argument has been proceeding very leisurely: "People don't often realize the little stratagem being played out under the guise of scientific objectivity."[36]

Jennifer: I don't like bacon anyway. It makes me thirsty, and then I drink a lot of milk, and milk gives me tummy-aches.

Kamens: Many people have milk allergies or sensitivities and are simply not aware of it.[37] Selection of a milk beverage can pose problems. If milk gives Jennifer an upset stomach, it would be better for her not to drink any.

Mom: But what about calcium and all the other nutrients in milk?

Kamens: We have been duped into thinking that milk is a perfect food. Dr. Robert S. Harris of M.I.T.'s nutrition biochemistry laboratory conducted a comparison study of very poor Mexican children and suburban children in Michigan. The Mexican children did not drink any milk at all. Surprisingly, the Mexican children had much better health scores than the Americans. They had much higher calcium levels.[38] Milk is not consumed in most cultures once a child is weaned from the breast. And the same is true of animals in the wild. Nor do these animals drink milk of *another* species.

Many researchers are convinced that milk would be a better product if it was not pasteurized or homogenized. Pasteurization reduces nutrients,[39] and homogenization has actually been shown to be harmful.[40, 41] Vitamin D added to milk may do more harm than good. One study shows that the added vitamin D activates an enzyme which contributes to heart disease, and that this process takes place because the milk has been pasteurized.[42] Dr. Lendon Smith, renowned pediatrician, calls milk "a dumb food."[43]

Robbie: Law #1 and Law #2. Processing and addition of harmful substances!

Mom: Are you saying that we should discontinue giving milk to the children?

Kamens: Again—we are discussing choices. Don't drink it or give it to your kids if the milk has an adverse effect. If homogenized milk is to be consumed at all, it should be simmered at 185°F for ten minutes. This inactivates the harmful enzyme (which, by the way, is not present in mother's milk). If you are eliminating milk from the diet, you should replace it with a healthful food product. Milk enhances a very poor diet, but does nothing much for an excellent diet. Fermented milk products (yogurt, kefir, buttermilk) can often be tolerated and digested more easily, even for those who are allergic and sensitive. And certified raw milk is a better product as it's less processed.

John: Whenever I have bread and butter, Mom makes me have a glass of milk with it. Now I can enjoy my bread and butter!

Dad: Since butter is made from milk, wouldn't that be harmful too?

Kamens: Butter does not contain the active enzyme, but ice cream does. Sorry about that! Whole and skim homogenized milk products also contain the enzyme.

John, the right kind of bread can make an excellent snack. When your Mom and Dad were little, they learned that bread was the "staff of life." Staff-of-life bread is very different from most of the bread available today. Real bread is made with whole grains, butter, milk, and eggs. Paul Stitt, a biochemist and food scientist, who draws on his many years of experience with the country's largest corporations, describes the depletion of bread quality this way:

> Wheat flour is one food which is especially ravaged by processing. In the refining process, more than half of each of the most essential nutrients are thrown away. The milling process destroys 40 percent of the chromium present in the whole grain, as well as 86 percent of the copper, 78 percent of the zinc, and 48 percent of the molybdenum. By the time the flour is completely refined, it has lost most of its phosphorus, iron, and thiamine, and a good deal of its niacin and riboflavin. Its crude fiber content has been cut down considerably as well. White flour has been plundered of most of its vitamin E, important oils and protein amino acids. Yet all of these nutrients are needed for a satisfied, healthy body. While whole wheat flour is one of the most nutritious foods, processing sees to it that the white flour found in most products is nutritionally worthless.[44]

After the wheat is stripped of its nutrients, the flour is bleached, the shortening is altered with sweetening agents (dextrose, refined sugar, and cheap corn syrup), the dough is stretched further with chemicals, and the yeast nutrients are synthetic.[45] The bread usually has a freshener added to it—not to preserve freshness, but to conceal staleness.[46]

Let's look at an ingredient listing of a popular bread. Note that enriched flour is one of the components. The term "enrichment" is a giveaway that the basic substances used have been depleted, and the manufacturer is trying to make up for this. If a bread has to be enriched, it's inferior to begin with. Only a few nutrients are replaced, and they are synthetic.[47, 48] William Dufty, famous journalist, writes in *Sugar Blues:* "If Dracula drains your blood with his teeth and gives you a vitamin B_{12} shot before he flies out the window, would you say you'd been had or enriched?"[49] At least one variety of bread contains powdered cellulose, which is a wood pulp byproduct.

Judy: Isn't that fiber?

Kamens: Yes, it is fiber, but we don't know if people can handle powdered cellulose (or wood pulp). Not enough studies have been done. It is suspected that wood pulp fiber does not react in a similar fashion as fiber found in foods naturally.

Jennifer: Law #2!

Kamens: Yes. We do know that excessive fiber of this kind may result in health problems because it causes loss of nutrients by binding minerals and interfering with the absorption of trace minerals. In natural foods, the necessary nutrients are present and accounted for.[50]

TABLE 19
THE GRAIN ROBBERY

Ingredient listing of popular bread: Water, flour, powdered cellulose, wheat gluten, wheat bran, whole wheat flour, brown sugar, yeast, salt, sugar, soy flour, calcium sulfate, whey, dough conditioners (may contain sodium stearoyl-2-lactylate, mono- and diglycerides, ethoxylated mono- and diglycerides, polysorbate 60, dicalcium phosphate, potassium bromate and/or barley malt, artificial flavor from (ferrous sulfate), niacin (A "B" Vitamin), thiamine, mononitrate (B_1), riboflavin (B_2), calcium propionate (to retard spoilage)

A study done in the home economics department at Arizona State University shows that natural fiber helps control blood-sugar levels, but that wood cellulose does not.[51] Blood-sugar levels are the key materials in your metabolism. You'll note in the ingredient listing of the bread that *whole-wheat flour* follows *enriched flour* and *powdered cellulose.* That means there is less of this product than of the preceding ingredients. Since brown sugar is farther down the list, you might wonder how this bread can be palatable with so little sweetener and so much wood pulp. If you skip an ingredient or two, you will note another sweetener: *sugar!*

Jennifer: Why don't they list both sugars together?

Kamens: The manufacturer is allowed to use as many as twelve or more different sweetening agents, and as long as they are not the same, they may be listed separately.[52] This is a ploy to detract from the fact that so much sugar is present in the product. If the two sugars were combined, the label would probably read, "water, *sugar,* enriched flour," and so on. . . .

"*Artificial Flavor*" is a term used for an endless number of substances, very many of them now being studied, but they are still allowed. And the vitamin listing does not reveal the fact that the vitamins are synthetic.[53]

Dad: A chemical is a chemical is a chemical. Aren't synthetic vitamins just as good as the real thing?

Kamens: Synthetic vitamins, even if identical in chemical structure to "natural" vitamins, do *not* have the same effect. Remember, they are not being consumed with their natural components. The nutrients that accompany "natural" vitamins (if they are in fact natural), may not be present in the synthetic substance. These components play an important role in your body's use of nutrients.[54] The term "natural" really should not be used. It is very confusing. Many vitamin and food products dubbed "natural" are anything but natural. And sometimes a synthetic vitamin is a better choice, or the only choice. (If the nutrient is needed in large quantities for therapeutic purposes, it might have to be synthetic.) The disturbing factor concerning the addition of synthetic vitamins to bread is that people are being misled. It's been shown, for example, that iron added to foods is very poorly absorbed.[55] Paul Stitt sums it up this way:

> By purchasing [enriched and vitamin fortified bread] you are being ripped off. . . . No wonder that, in one research project, two thirds of the rats kept on a ninety-day diet of enriched white bread died before the experiment was finished.[56]

Dad: I read an article stating that whole-wheat bread affects mineral absorption.

Mom: And the whole-wheat bread in the supermarket has preservatives in it!

Sherry: I don't like whole-wheat bread.

Kamens: Let's deal with your comments one at a time. Some minerals in wheat are *incompletely available*. That means they are not utilized by your body. But this is true of some nutrients in almost all foods. The troublemaker in wheat is *phosphate*, which may affect phosphorus, calcium, magnesium, iron, copper, and zinc. Dr. Davis, of the Clayton Foundation Biochemical Institute, tells us that the human digestive system can slowly adapt to some of the effects of phytin (the salt of the phytic acid found in wheat). In addition, yeast and leavening of bread modify the detrimental effects of the phytic acid. Sprouting of seeds also destroys phytic acid. So sprouted-grain breads and wheat products leavened by yeast are superior to those that are unleavened or leavened mechanically or leavened by baking powder.[57] Nature has a way of balancing things, if only we give it a chance. By the way, vitamin C increases the absorption of iron from whole-grain breads. The ascorbic acid actually breaks down the iron and fiber bond.[58]

Mrs. Palmer, your comment about the preservatives in whole wheat breads is important. There are many implications. Because whole grains tend to get rancid quickly, commercial manufacturers often lean heavily on additives. A famous nutritionist has made the statement that if he had no other choice, he would select supermarket *white* bread in preference to the whole wheat because of rancidity problems. Since very few commercial breads are additive-free, you have to look at the small print on the package. And be on the look-out for advertising jargon. The statement "no preservatives" does not necessarily mean there are no other additives.

Sherry, people who do not like whole-grain products find them "strong" tasting. But since most taste preferences are *learned*, they can also be *unlearned*. Those who responded negatively to whole-grain foods once-upon-a-time, find white bread too "mushy" after making the transition to the more natural "whole" varieties. In fact, using the touch system when buying bread is helpful. If you can "play piano" on the loaves, forget it.

John: And watch out for the preservatives. The bread lasts forever—only the eater disappears.

Mom: So what do we do? Is there any bread that *is* respectable?

Kamens: Try your local natural food store. In addition to the possibility of finding just the product you are looking for, you have another opportunity: Many people who shop in these stores are very knowledgeable about the best source for this or that. However, with a family as large as yours, why not consider baking your own bread? You have so many helping hands.

Dad: I might give it a try. I like to bake.

Mom: But doesn't whole-wheat flour get just as rancid in your own kitchen as anyplace else?

Kamens: Grains remain dormant as long as they are left intact—left in their whole, unground state. Buy a bag of wheatberries and grind your own flour *as needed.* (Grinders are inexpensive.) The bonus? No rancidity. No loss of nutrients. Astounding flavor. Unbelievable aroma. Each of the children should take turns with the preparation, or have specific chores to be rotated every week.

Sherry: We'd be just like the Waltons!

Kamens: Smaller families bake a number of loaves at a time, and freeze the bread. There are nutrient losses in the freezing process, but home-baked bread, even if frozen, is far superior to most breads available—especially the commercial varieties. And look at the possibility of money savings by going back to more basic food preparation:

Jennifer: What about our *cereal?* I bet it's okay, because Mom doesn't let us get the kind with sugar.

Kamens: You will find many surprises if you look at the labels on most cereal boxes—even the ones without sugar coatings. (Note the sugar

TABLE 20
GRINDING DOWN THE COST

Relative Costs for 1,000 Calories of Whole Grain

Form of grain	Cost per 1000 calories
Bulk grain	$.05
Whole-wheat flour	.15
Bread or cereal	.50

From "Wheat and Nutrition," by Dr. Donald R. Davis, department of chemistry, Clayton Foundation Biochemical Institute of the University of Texas at Austin, published in *Nutrition Today* 16 (September/October 1981): 22–25.

content of cereals in Table 5.) A few cereals advertised as being made of "natural, healthful" products contain large quantities of refined sugar. For cereal packaging, the grains are flaked, crinkled, cracked, popped, puffed, shredded, rounded, colored, textured, and the finished product is a food from which important nutrients are subtracted, just like the whole grain of the bread. The natural structure of the cereal grain is altered. Once again, the more processing, the fewer nutrients.[59]

Mom: Oh, but the cereals are so convenient and easy and appetizing. Doesn't that count for something?

Kamens: Your question implies that natural foods are inconvenient and unappetizing, and nothing could be further from the truth. The fact is, preparing your own supply of cold cereals not only reduces cost (you could make enough for several months), but the homemade variety has more nutrients than you will ever find in the colorful packages.

John: I love *hot* cereals.

Kamens: Going the route of hot cereals is easier because there are good choices on the supermarket shelf. For wheat cereal, select the *whole* grains type, not the bleached, white varieties from which the bran and germ have been removed. (The germ contains vitamins, oils, and protein, and the bran supplies minerals, fiber, and more protein and vitamins.[60]) Oatmeal is packaged with the bran and germ intact, making commercial oatmeal a good choice.[61]

Robbie: Even instant oatmeal?

Kamens: Think about it for a moment. What would make a product instant?[62]

Robbie: Back to the drawing board: Laws of Choice #1 and #2. I suppose there has to be another processing step to make it instant.

Kamens: Instant *anything* means:
1) the addition of an unwanted additive, or
2) precooking, or
3) more processing.

John: I like oatmeal with lots of margarine.

Kamens: Margarine is a man-made artificial product, lacking the nutrients of butter.[63, 64] If you want to lubricate your cereal, butter is a better choice.

Judy: But isn't margarine less fattening than butter?

Kamens: Margarine has the same amount of fat as butter. As a matter of fact, margarine contains an unnatural distorted fat. Margarine also has artificial butter-like flavor, odor and color, plus chemically flavored protectors and preservatives.[65] Compare the label of margarine with non-dyed butter, and you decide which you want to eat.

Judy: Well, another dieting trick goes down the drain. Is there anything less fattening than butter that I can put in my cereal? I try not to have milk in cereal, either.

Kamens: Try apple sauce, apple juice, diced fresh pineapple, or a little yogurt. Sliced banana does the trick, too.

Sherry: Why do they sell foods that are not good for you?

John: To make money, silly.

Robbie: It's not illegal to sell it.

Kamens: Profit is a major motive. Some products are developed simply because there is a byproduct to dispose of, or new markets to explore. When any medical research is disclosed, however premature, the food industry jumps on the bandwagon as an excuse to promote their products, or create new ones. Interpretations of biological research have become very distorted. The basic principle of whole nourishment has gone by the wayside. As stated earlier, nourishment is a *process*, and cannot be regarded in single cause and effect relationships.

There's the story of the researcher who enters his laboratory one morning and finds that dozens of cheese-baited mouse traps all over the room each contain one dead mouse. He calls the F.D.A., and reports, "I have proved conclusively that cheese causes death in mice."

Jennifer: But some things that are bad are good. Like salt. It's bad, but you need it. Right?

Kamens: You do need *sodium*, Jennifer, but it's unlikely that you would ever have a sodium deficiency. Sodium abounds in natural foods, and it's added to processed foods.[66]

The chances are you have much more sodium in your diet than you require. Salt has a way of creeping into your daily food one way or another. Comparing the sodium content in a few foods demonstrates that there is far less sodium in the more natural food products.

Robbie: Enough with breakfast. How about lunch?

Judy: I'm eating out.

John: I have to eat lunch in school.

TABLE 21
SALT TALKS

Food Item	Serving	Sodium (mgs)
Total brand cereal	1 oz.	415
Puffed Wheat cereal	1 oz.	2
English muffin	1	633
Whole-wheat toast	1	264
Italian dressing (bottled)	1 tbsp.	314
Oil and vinegar	1 tbsp.	—

From "How Salt Creeps into Daily Diets," by Bonnie Liebman, in *Nutrition Action*, April 1981, p. 5.

Jennifer: I have lunch in a bag.

Kamens: One in three Americans buys lunch, and an increasing handful brown-bag it. The quality of food available in most restaurants is not quite up to par, even if the restaurant is elegant. The correlation between diet and disease is no longer theory. We now know that minor disorders like acne, and major ills such as cancer, can be diet-related.[67] Therefore, *every meal should be of optimal quality.*

Judy: Doesn't the FDA check out all the restaurants?

Kamens: The FDA has a rough job. There is such widespread use and abuse of so many products, it is almost impossible to police all of them. Government agencies cannot be depended on for full protection.[68] It took sixteen years for one pesticide to be banned from the time it was first recognized as dangerous.[69] Manufacturer deceit is demonstrated in the canned apple juice scandal. Several brands of apple juice, labeled "sugar free" were recently tested. Of those studied, at least six had significant amounts of refined sugar which had been added.[70]

Jennifer: Well, Mom gives us sandwiches for lunch anyway. It's usually cold cuts. But now that we know about nitrites. . . .

Kamens: Luncheon meats are very popular sandwich fillings. The Center for Science in the Public Interest has rated foods according to nutrient quality. Bologna is down at the bottom of the chart, liver is way up at the top, and dog food some place in the middle.[71]

Dad: Do the luncheon meats get such a low rating because of their nitrites?

Kamens: Luncheon meats are highly processed. They are often made from meats of the lowest possible grade, and have artificial colors and flavors.[72]

John: Since we can't have cold cuts anymore, I would take peanut butter sandwiches. That is, if I could take lunch.

Kamens: The most popular lunch spread! Many commercial peanut butters are heavily endowed with sugar. Some have molasses in addition to sugar, plus chemical emulsifiers to prevent the oil from separating and extend the shelf life of the product. The germ or heart of the peanut is often removed in processing. The germ is the little bump you see when you separate the two parts of the nut. This part of the peanut will spoil quickly. Of course, it is also the part of the peanut that is very high in nutrient value. Most commercial peanut butter just isn't the healthful food product the manufacturers would have you believe it is.[73]

Robbie: Why is sugar so bad for us?

Kamens: Remember Law #1? The more processed, the less nutrient value. Sugar is just about the most processed food there is. Ninety percent of the original sugar cane or sugar beet is removed in processing. Sugar has been accused of being a contributing factor in cancer, heart disease, diabetes, reduced ability to fight infection—and acne.[74, 75]

John: Hey! Wait a minute! Apples have sugar, and apples are good for us. So why can't we add the sugar to cereals?

Kamens: Dr. Ross Hume Hall, renowned nutritional biochemist of Canada, tells us: "The sugar [in your cereal] is refined sucrose. The sugar in apples is a mixture of fructose, glucose and sucrose, imbedded in a fibrous matrix together with other nutrients designed to accompany the sugars. The insulin and metabolic responses from eating apples and from eating naked sucrose differ greatly."[76]

Mom: Except for morning cereal, we really don't use the sugar bowl.

Kamens: Sugar has a way of hiding. It's highly absorbent. There is refined sugar in ketchup, yogurt, juices, instant breakfasts, chewing gum, cough drops, mouthwash, pickles, chewable vitamins, and there is even sugar in salt.

Sherry: Sugar in salt? That sounds funny.

Kamens: Look at the label on the salt box. It probably says, "dextrose."[77] Many lunchboxes contain desserts with large quantities of sugar, and also endless chemicals—lists so long they hardly fit on the packages (even if the print is minuscule). Do you really want to eat these substances that are so new to human experience and, by the way, totally foreign to the animal kingdom?

John: My health teacher said if we eat foods from the four food groups, we'll have balanced meals.
Kamens: Do you remember what the food groups are?
John: Sure. Fruits and vegetables, grains, dairy, and meat.
Kamens: Before we tampered with food, the four-food-group concept worked. Unfortunately, a fast-food meal of a hamburger on a roll, with french fries and cole slaw, plus a shake, fits the four-food groupings.
Judy: That sounds good to me.
Kamens: Yes, doesn't it? And you know, it could be delicious *and* nutritious—if the rolls were whole grain; the hamburgers free of additives and not quite so fatty; if the potatoes were fried in fresh oil at lower temperatures; and finally, if the drinks were extracted from natural fruit rather than concoctions of sugar, caffeine, color additives, etc.
Judy: By the time you leave, I think the only thing left in the fridge will be cottage cheese and the light bulb.
Kamens: Sometimes, when you are aware of good nutrition, you seek foods you *think* are healthful, like cottage cheese.
Mom: Oh no, what's wrong with cottage cheese?
Kamens: Nothing. That is, nothing with cottage cheese per se—but—the curds are often washed in a chemical that hastens factory procedures; butter flavor may be added; salt added; dyes, preservatives, bleaches, stabilizers, mold inhibitors. Cottage cheese is highly perishable and, like hundreds of other food products, it's listed as a "standard of identity." This means that as long as the manufacturer follows the limits of set recipes, the ingredients need not be listed.[78] With little exception, nowhere on the label of cottage cheese will you find a complete listing of ingredients. To add to the confusion, the manufacturer has the option of listing only some of the ingredients. Again—you are not aware that the listing may be partial.[79]
Judy: I repeat my question. What's left to eat?

TABLE 22
STANDARDS OF IDENTITY: WHAT'S IN IT FOR YOU?

Chief Groups of Standardized Foods Not Requiring Labeling

Cocoa	Milk
Macaroni	Canned fruits
Cheeses	Cream
Processed cheese	Fruit juices
Flour	Tomato products
Chocolate	Preserves
Farina	Jellies
Mayonnaise	Cornmeal
Bread	Salad dressings
Ice cream	

From Federal Drug Administration, Hicksville, New York.

Kamens: At its *simplest,* a juicy piece of fruit, a savory wedge of cheese, a bowl of crunchy nuts, a thick slice of chewy raisin-speckled whole-grain bread, a crackly peanut butter cookie. At its most *splendid,* mouth-watering cornucopias that are as diverse as they are appealing.

Does the prospect of an Oriental dish comprised of brown rice and tamari, laced with crispy bits of stir-fried peppers, celery, mushrooms, onions, and zucchini—delicately seasoned with ginger and garlic—set your salivary glands in motion? This is real food. This is "cuisine santé," the cuisine of health. This is food that excites. You are presently enticed by salt and sugar and greasy fat. A range of tastes inherent in food itself, with overtones of herbs and spices to enhance, offer sheer sensual pleasure. When real food stimulates taste buds, when you recognize the inner flavor of food, the *soul* of food, you will show the door to what you now call food, or to meals you now consume.

Robbie: I have a feeling my days as a junk-food freak are numbered.

Kamens: The different dishes multiply when you begin to learn the culinary skills of preparing textured salads, profusions of vegetables, ambrosias, marvelous course-grained feasts—using the season's bounty plus your imagination. Every meal is like an apple off another tree, whether it's breakfast, lunch, or dinner. [See the recipe section for help.]

Dad: All those plant-based foods! What about complete protein? The need for amino acids in the right proportions? Would a large salad alone offer that?

Kamens: Good question. There are several ways that vegetable protein transforms into amino acid patterns—patterns that comply with human needs.

1) There is assurance of having enough of the amino acids that are in limited supply by consuming *large quantities* of vegetables and grains. An Oriental might eat a pound of rice a day.

2) Adding small amounts of *animal protein* to the vegetable or grain diet will turn the protein trick. Examples are: A glass of milk with bread; a little milk in cereal; yogurt as a dressing for salad; salad garnished with strips of meat (chicken, etc.). In Asian cultures, meat or poultry is used as a condiment. This way you *use* rather than *lose* the vegetable protein. A boost of high-quality protein from animal sources (as found in an egg) has been shown to result in superior health for a strict vegetarian.

3) Many cereals and legumes combine well to form complete protein. The *combining of complementary foods* is widely practiced. Illustrations are: peanut butter and bread, split pea soup and crackers, rice and beans, tortillas and beans, cereal and sesame seeds, yams and beans. All these "twosomes" combine to make complete protein. One plant food compensates for the other's deficiencies.[80, 81]

Robbie: I learned that although we represent only seven percent of the world's population, we eat thirty percent of the world's supplies of animal protein.

Kamens: Yes. Orientals eat very little meat. We consume thirty times as much meat as the Japanese, and sixty-six times as much as the average Asian. The most expensive part of the human diet anywhere in the world is protein from animal sources. Three-quarters of a cup of beans and two cups of rice have the same amount of usable protein as a ten-ounce steak. The steak costs four times as much as the beans and rice.[82]

Dad: One of my colleagues talks about super-foods. Is there really any such thing?

Kamens: Super-foods offer more nutrients per serving than average foods. A case in point is the avocado. It has just about all the known nutrients. An added gift comes from its thick skin—it doesn't require spraying.[83] Sprouts, another super-food, should embellish every meal. It's so easy to sprout, and this is one way of getting fresh vegetables, inexpensively—vegetables growing in your own kitchen right up to the moment you use them in your recipes. Alfalfa sprouts have been known to increase resistance to disease. The tiny seeds grow fast and furiously, are among the easiest of the sprouts to grow, and for many, are the most delicious.[84]

Mom: Could you suggest sandwich ideas—quick, easy sandwiches?

Kamens: How about a sliced egg stuffed into a pita pouch, augmented with cucumber and/or tomato and onion with sugar-free and additive-free mayonnaise? Line the pouch with lettuce or some other green. Tasty! Quick! Delicious! Healthful! Combine super-foods—an avocado-sprout sandwich on whole grain bread.

A master stroke is to prepare more than the usual quantity of chicken or fish for dinner, anticipating leftovers. (With the appetite of this large family, you will have to hide the surplus.) Cold chicken with slices of apple in a mustard-lined pita pouch is superb. Once you've tasted homemade fish salad, nevermore will your electric opener dig its teeth into cans of tuna. [See Lunch Box Logic menus in the recipe section.]

Mom: Why do I *still* feel like a fish in troubled waters—swimming upstream? I feel threatened.

Kamens: We all feel that way at first because anything unfamiliar appears to be difficult. In *Nutrition, Behavior and Change,* the authors state:

> Resistance to change is normal. Most of us are creatures of habit; the easiest way to do things is the way we have always done them. Experimentation with the unfamiliar is a stimulating challenge for some but creates discomfort and insecurity for others. Sometimes action may not be immediately applicable to personal practice.[85]

Just a little planning at the beginning, and "new" becomes routine. It is unwise to make too many changes at once. You will accomplish miracles if you plan *one change a month.* Start by adding good foods before removing harmful ones. Don't take anything away until you have wholesome substitutes. It has been said that if you don't put the effort into health, you'll have to put it into illness. The message is that everyone has a right to health, but that your *health is your own responsibility.*

Dad: Isn't a total diet of all healthful foods very expensive?

Kamens: Processed foods are expensive because the cost of packaging and preparation are included in the final price. Consider potatoes as an example: Locally grown potatoes are about *20 cents* a pound. If the potatoes are shipped from California, the price almost doubles. If the potatoes are packaged as french fries in a box, you may pay *79 cents* a pound. Canned? *85 cents* a pound. Large bag of potato chips? *$2.20!* Small bag? *$2.90!* Pringles brand (chips in a tennis ball can)? *$2.50!* Potato sticks in a can? *$3.30!* And there is one more point: *Food that doesn't nourish you is expensive.*

Dad: Well, I'm impressed. . . . Now that you've gotten us through breakfast and lunch, how about the rest of the day? That's when *I* usually have problems.

Kamens: When the pace slackens at the end of the day there is a tendency to clip the wings of good eating habits. There are tips, however, on how to enjoy evening snacks.

Mom: Okay, but first tell me: What should I prepare for dinner?

Kamens: As the one in charge of culinary activities, the greatest burden is yours. You do want the next generation to enjoy good health, with whole, real foods as part of everyday living. *You* have to work a little harder as you shift gears. When your children are homemakers, the "new" regimens will be part of their heritage. You are giving them a very precious gift. So, on with dinner. Of course, the food producer tries to make it easy by offering many already prepared foods.

Sherry: You mean like TV dinners?

Kamens: Yes, but many nutrients are lost when foods are gassed, waxed, dyed, soaked, peeled, overcooked—processes used when food is frozen, canned, and bottled, and then stored, and recooked. Food canned or frozen no longer has its original nutrient content.[86, 87] If food sits around for several months without benefit of these processing steps, it will not look, smell or taste like food fit for human consumption.

Dad: My grandmother always ridiculed us for not buying fresh vegetables. We thought she was old-fashioned.

Kamens: She might have been critical either because she chose not to change her own ways, or from wisdom handed down to her. She probably understood exactly what was happening.

Judy: Is it really so terrible if some foods don't have all the nutrients

TABLE 23
CANNERY COUNTDOWN

Percent of Nutrient Losses in the Canning Process

Vegetable	B_6	A	Thiamin	Riboflavin	Niacin	C
Green Beans	50	51.7	62.5	63.6	40	78.9
Carrots	53.6	9.1	66.7	60	33.3	75
Corn	0	32.5	80	58.3	47.1	58.3
Green Peas	68.8	29.7	74.2	64.3	69	66.7

From Robert S. Harris, ed., and Endel Karmas, ed., *Nutritional Evaluation of Food Processing*, second ed. (Westport, CT: The AVI Publishing Co., Inc., 1977), p. 229.

they started with? Don't we eat enough foods through the day to make up for it?

Kamens: Would you want to travel in a plane that has a few parts missing? If the plane is under stress, those missing parts may be crucial. Sometimes the imperfect functioning of one mechanism causes stress on another mechanism. The same is true of the human body.

Before World War II, commercially prepared foods were produced by the same methods used at home. Today, the foods you buy are the result of very sophisticated technology, The commercial techniques employed since the 1940's could only be duplicated in factories. Let's use pizza as an example. The grains for the crust are highly refined—the bran and germ of the wheat have been removed. The cheese could be and usually is artificial. The tomato paste and even the sausage are often synthetic too. If the pizza is frozen, it's cooked a second time when defrosted. When you purchase pizza in a restaurant, you have no way of knowing the pedigree of that pizza. (Restaurant foods are often frozen nowadays.)[88] You forget—or don't even know—that some of the foods you consume should not be called foods.

The food distributors have arranged for endless choices of accessory "helpers" to enhance your meal. These products are often woven with additives, coloring agents, preservatives, buffers, neutralizers, moisture-control agents, flavorings, bleaching agents, maturing agents, etc.

Mom: But "helpers" do "help" the budget.

TABLE 24A
THE MAKING OF A PIZZA: 20TH CENTURY—PART 1

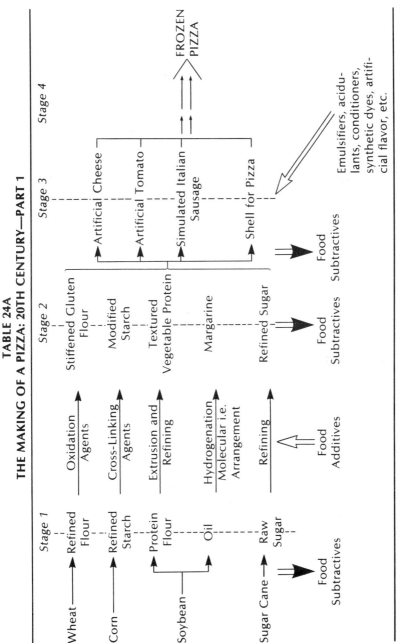

From Ross Hume Hall, "The Making of a Pizza," 1978, *En-Trophy Institute for Advanced Study*, Vol. 1, No. 3 (March–April, 1978), p. 5

TABLE 24B
THE MAKING OF A PIZZA: 20TH CENTURY—PART 2

Frozen Pizza Ingredients

CRUST: Enriched bleached flour (wheat flour, malted barley flour, niacin, reduced iron, potassium bromate, thiamine mononitrate, riboflavin), water, soy flour, yeast, salt, soybean oil, monocalcium phosphate, sodium bicarbonate, dextrose, calcium propionate dough conditioners (sodium stearoyl-2-lactylate, succinylated and distilled monoglycerides, sodium metabisulfite), whey powder

SAUCE: Tomato purée, sugar, salt, spieces, garlic oil, granulated onion, natural flavors, xanthan gum

TOPPINGS: Cheddar cheese, low-moisture part-skim mozzarella cheese, dehydrated onions, spices, dehydrated parsley

From: Label on frozen pizza package

Kamens: There are inexpensive primary foods that are fabulous supporters. You can extend hamburger meat with mashed, sprouted garbanzo beans. This will reduce cost, double quantity, and triple nutrient value. Or follow Jane Kinderlehrer's advice in her marvelous book *Confessions of a Sneaky Organic Cook* (Rodale Press). Jane suggests the addition of organ meats as extenders. She says that 2 pounds of *chuck*, mixed with 1 pound of *heart* gives her 3 pounds of meat at half the price. Before you moan and groan about eating organ meats, we can only say, "Try it, you'll like it." In fact, Jane's son asked her to give the hamburger recipe to his wife, not ever knowing what the ingedients were. He just remembered that Mom's hamburgers were the best!

TABLE 25
THE HELPLESS HAMBURGER

Ingredients for Hamburger Helper: Enriched macaroni, dried cheddar cheese, modified cornstarch, partially hydrogenated soybean oil, dried tomato, salt, buttermilk, sugar, hydrolized vegetable protein and other natural flavoring, dried onion, dried corn syrup, disodium phosphate (for smooth sauce), dried garlic, sodium caseinate (milk protein), citric acid (for flavor), dipotassium phosphate (for smooth sauce), FD&C yellow no. 5 and other artificial color, color and freshness preserved by sodium sulfite and BHA.

Judy: I think I'm beginning to understand the definition of primary foods. What about skim milk? My skin breaks out easily, so I've been avoiding whole milk because of its fat content. Have I been doing the right thing?

Kamens: Judy, what are the laws?

Judy: The more processed, the fewer nutrients and stay away from additives.

Kamens: Can you answer your own question?

Judy: I'm not sure.

Kamens: To cut the "skinnyness" of real skim milk, emulsifiers (such as tapioca) may be used. Without an emulsifier, fat-free milk would be unpalatable.

The removal of fat from milk makes it an unbalanced food. Fat is necessary for the proper assimilation of calcium, one of the reasons dietitians recommend milk to begin with. Skim milk is not a balanced food. It is not a *primary* food. And again, many people are allergic to milk or have milk intolerance, and don't even know it.

And if you're still not convinced about cholesterol, several experiments (studies of Masai tribesmen in Africa, experiments at Penn State University, and human testing at Vanderbilt University) show that cholesterol levels *drop* as milk consumption increases. The researchers have actually isolated a substance in whole milk that inhibits cholesterol production in the liver.

Judy: Isn't there some kind of "safe" list that the FDA has put together—a list that advises what's okay and what isn't?

Kamens: You are referring to the GRAS roll-call. GRAS means "generally recognized as safe." The list was compiled in 1958, but there is almost complete lack of testing of the generally-recognized-as-safe postings.[89] Testing has begun slowly. However, over 31 million Americans are allergic to the tiniest amount of some of the chemicals in food.[90]

Robbie: So what *are* we having for dinner?

Kamens: Millions of years of use of natural, whole foods has determined your ability to metabolize—or utilize—those foods. And these are the foods you will do best on.[91] Let's have a dinner of *whole* foods, primary foods.

John: That sounds like vegetables. Do I have to stay for dinner?

Robbie: Hey, John—it's either shelf life or *your* life!

Kamens: You know we don't mean opening a can of peas and carrots. We don't like those either. There are varieties of grains and vegetables that can be prepared in many different, interesting and even exotic recipes, such as barley with pearl onions and bits of carrot; peppers stuffed with millet, topped with cheese; rice casseroles, etc. In fact, one-half of the world's population considers rice a basic food.[92] However, when brown rice is milled to make white or polished rice, nutrient values are diminished.[93]

Sherry: Law #1!

Kamens: Law #1. Severe nutritional deficiencies are produced when the larger part of the diet is comprised of the "modern" polished white rice because it is so overmilled.[94]

Mom: Are we excluding meat entirely? And are we limiting chicken?

Robbie: Dad always says someone should cross a chicken with a centipede, so we get drumsticks for everyone, because chicken legs are our favorites.

Kamens: Meat, along with fowl and fish and eggs are primary foods that don't require labeling. These are foods your great grandparents ate. But much of the meat available today is no longer "pure." Many animals live indoors in crowded cages or stalls. The cramped conditions induce stress, which in turn encourages disease. Drugs and chemicals are standard fare for these animals. The result? Poor-quality meat and chicken containing chemical residues.[95]

Mom: What about *raw* foods?

Kamens: Every meal should include raw foods, or one entire meal could be a raw food meal. Salads, of course, are excellent vehicles for raw foods. The salad you have for lunch can be quite different from the salad you have for dinner. There are galaxies of choices. One caution: Don't use head lettuce. Head lettuce, or iceberg lettuce as it is also called, is easy to pack, ship and store, but it's also the least nutritious, and the most sprayed. Sometimes as many as seven or more doses are applied.[96] Romaine lettuce contains many times the vitamin A, and much more calcium and iron. Butterheads and other soft-head, green lettuce types contain two or three times the vitamin A, calcium, and iron as the commercial favorite head lettuce.[97, 98]

Jennifer: When do we get to dessert?

Kamens: Right now! What could be easier than a beautiful fruit bowl on the table? Fruit may help you get rid of unwanted contaminants. It has been shown that strontium 90, a radioactive fall-out, is forced out of the body by the pectin found in apples and lemons.[99, 100]

Robbie: What about desserts sweetened with honey?

Sherry: Honey is just a little bit good, so it's not nutritious, right?

John: Honey is *very* nutritious.

Judy: Honey is *not* good.

Kamens: There appears to be a lot of confusion about honey. Honey is twice as sweet as sugar, so only half as much serves the same purpose as sugar. In addition, it does have some minerals. But it is still very high in carbohydrates. The "purist" nutrition advocate uses very little honey. It's a good sweetener to use while the family is in the process of food changes. Let's call it a "transition" food.

Dad: Apparently in the land of milk and honey, we'll do fine if we stay away from milk and honey.

Kamens: Remember that sugar in fruit is digested *slowly.* It's not dumped into your bloodstream as quickly as refined sugar. Therefore, an apple is not digested as quickly as ice cream. Hunger pangs will attack in a shorter time span after eating ice cream than after eating an apple. Ice cream contains refined sugar; the apple contains natural sugar.[101]

Mom: We always get the "munchies" in the evening, and we nibble our way through the last hours of the day.

Kamens: Most Americans do not stop eating when dinner is over. That's when the fun begins! But making more healthful choices need not diminish the pleasures. Nuts and seeds satisfy "munchies." Again—there are myriad selections offering a range of good nutrients.

Judy: What about nuts that are already shelled? You know, the kind that are packaged or canned?

Robbie: Dummy, remember Law #1—and probably Law #2. Right?

Kamens: Yes, Robbie, right. The more processed, the fewer nutrients—even for nuts. Commercially packaged nuts are usually highly salted. Salt is added to many foods for gusto.

Salt is also used to conceal stale or rancid flavors.[102] Too much salt causes lower potassium and higher sodium levels, which is a reversal of the natural ratio.[103] The sodium you eat affects your potassium. Potassium is a mineral needed for *every* cell in your body. It is especially important for good athletic function.[104] The flipflop proportions created by eating salted foods (more salt and less potassium) is a distortion of biological relationships, and is considered to be one of the causes of heart disease.[105, 106]

Some people are highly susceptible, and become hypertensive with small amounts of salt. Others don't react, or do so only after a long period of time. We don't really know how many people are salt-sensitive, but we do know that an estimated 17 percent of adult Americans develop high blood pressure on a daily salt intake of only 3 to 6 grams. This reflects maladaptations that start in childhood. (The Senate Select Committee for Human Nutrition has stated that the average American consumes 16 grams of salt per day.[107]) Dr. Henry Blackburn, department of physiological hygiene of the University of Minnesota, sums it up:

> High levels of sodium intake are created and maintained by the introduction of salt to infant foods, by the heavy salting used in food processing, by the highly salted snack foods, and by food traditions. To illustrate how salt is hidden in ordinary foods: french fries at a popular fast food restaurant have less sodium than any of its burgers, egg dishes, milk shakes, or apple pies. . . . Food processing in the U.S. drives out much of the naturally occurring potassium just as it adds salt.[108]

Sodium is only one of the problems that comes along for the ride with packaged nuts. Many pecans are marked "fine." This is a Madison Avenue term meaning "select." It really means "tampered with." Can you think of other similar Madison Avenue words?

Mom: "Choice"; "new."

Dad: "Enriched."

Judy: "Superior."

Robbie: "Deluxe."

Jennifer: "Fortified."

John: "Improved."

Sherry: "Snap-Crackle-Pop."

Kamens: And the terms "natural" and "wholesome" and "nutritious" are used to "dupe" the poor unknowing consumer. In the case of the pecans, "fine" means bleached and polished—polished with shellac. The shellac and the bleach may leach into the nuts. Natural untreated pecans (which are really the "fine" ones) are not shiny or uniform in color.[109] A yogurt bar claims to have more "balanced nutrition" than

TABLE 26
RATIOS: RATIONAL AND IRRATIONAL
(SODIUM AND POTASSIUM)

Food (100-gram portion)	Sodium (mgs)	Potassium (mgs)
Rational		
Apples	1	110
Bananas	1	370
Peas	0.9	380
Potatoes	3	244
Irrational		
Canned peas	230	180
Frankfurters	1100	230
Cornflakes	660	165
White bread	570	205

From Dietary Goals for the U.S., second ed., prepared by the Select Committee on Nutrition and Human Needs, U.S. Senate, U.S. Government Printing Office, Washington, 1977; and Benjamin H. Ershoff, "Effects of Dietary Sodium Ratio in the Treatment of Hypertension," Journal of Applied Nutrition, Vol. 33, No. 2 (1981).

an 8-ounce portion of yogurt. Since fat and sugar are the main ingredients in the bar (yogurt places fifth), how can the company make this claim? Well, it's based on an assumed definition of "balanced nutrition." The manufacturer says balanced nutrition means a lot of vitamins and minerals, and they disregard other substances in the product. Do you think this is "balanced nutrition"?[110]

Another company advertises that its variety of potato chips has calories equivalent to those in a cup of milk, and has the same amount of salt as found in two slices of bread. Balanced nutrition?

It's fun to sit around after dinner with a nutcracker and a bowl of nuts. Another delightful after-dinner snack is the sunflower seed. A pocket full of polly seeds is a pocket full of power. Columbus discovered America *and* the sunflower seed.

Judy: I thought the Russians discovered sunflower seeds.

Kamens: The Russians eat a lot of sunflower seeds. Columbus took the sunflower seeds back to Europe and today, they are eaten mostly abroad![111] The Russians tell us that the pectin in sunflower seeds is a "detoxifying" substance: a substance that helps our bodies get rid of contaminants.[112]

Sherry: Does this mean we can't have popcorn anymore?

Kamens: Popcorn is not on the restricted list. But don't use the dyed, already buttered and salted kind. It's fun to pop the corn. Set out a bowl of freshly made popcorn and a bowl of sliced fruit and see how quickly the platters are wiped clean.

Dad: Judy and I have a real sweet tooth. I'm not sure the fruit and nut routine will satisfy us.

Kamens: It's hard to believe, but people who have made the food changes will tell you that you do lose the unnatural sweet tooth when there are better choices available. Desires for "sweet" and "salt" are acquired. Mixtures of nuts and seeds and dried fruit can be combined in an infinite number of ways. They usually satisfy the craving for something sweet. So do attractive platters of fresh fruit and yogurt. Pineapple, banana, and papaya can be used as sweetening agents in many recipes

Five top-selling candy bars were recently found to have traces of cancer-causing chemicals. Candy becomes far less appetizing when you learn about "Filth Guidelines" set up by the FDA.[113]

TABLE 27
FILTH GUIDELINES

Filth Tolerances for Unavoidable Defects

Product	Acceptable Limits
Chocolate	60 microscopic insect fragments per 100 grams
Cocoa Powder	75 microscopic insect fragments per 50 grams
Cocoa Beans	4% mold or 4% insect infestation by count

From *Eating May be Hazardous to Your Health,* by Jacqueline Verrett and Jean Carper, pp. 221–22.

Sherry: OOOHHH. I'm not eating chocolate again.

Robbie: Wanna bet?

Judy: Why are such extreme things done to foods? I mean, there are snacks at the supermarket that are really weird. Tasty, but weird. I realize now these products are not real food.

Kamens: What do you think your great grandparents would say if they entered a supermarket and saw Ring Dings and Crunch 'N Munch and Suzy Q's . . .

Judy: And Sno-Balls and Yodels and Bugles.

Robbie: And Fudge Mates and Twinkies and Trix.

Jennifer: And Pringles and Yankee Doodles and Franken Berries.

John: And Switzers and Twizzlers and Chuckles.

Sherry: And Bravo and Rold Gold and Fiddle Faddle.

Dad: My grandma would say, *"Fiddlesticks!"*

Mom: Never mind Grandma! How do my children know about these so-called foods? *I* don't buy them!

Kamens: Five cents' worth of wheat or corn can be sold for $2.00 in factory-made forms. Obviously, it is more profitable to create super-packaged, appealing, convenience snacks.

Judy: The boys I date are into beer drinking. How dangerous is the occasional beer-bout? Isn't there some nutrient value in beer?

Kamens: There is some food value in beer beyond its alcohol calories, but it is so slight that one ounce of bread contains more nutrients (including vitamins), than a bottle of beer.[114] Beer may contain a preservative, a foam stabilizer, an acid to adjust the pH (the acid-alkaline ratios), a water corrective, an antibiotic and chemical fermenting agents. Beer is also on the list of those foods especially high in lead from processing equipment.[115]

John: We didn't go into detail about my favorite snack: cheese.

Kamens: Cheese may be a good protein snack, provided it isn't overused. Most cheeses, even the imported, have coloring agents added. If the color is not mixed with the cheese itself, these cosmetic additives are included in the rind.[116] But there are natural cheeses on the market.

Dad: Ah! What could possibly take the place of a pizza and a cola drink?

Kamens: How about some carbonated water mixed with fruit juice? This kind of drink has a zing, and it's thirst quenching. No additives or

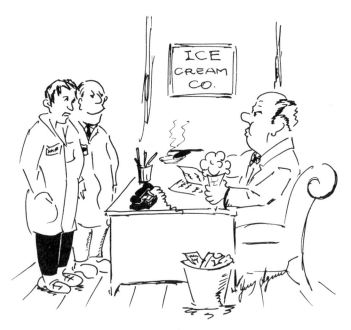

Don't worry about the dairy strike. It's been a long time since we used real farm ingredients in our ice cream.

caffeine here for allergic dermatitis reactions. Instead of chemicals you are now consuming protein, bioflavonoids, vitamins, minerals—real nutrients.[117] Homemade pizza is so simple: pita bread, tomato sauce with seasonings, topped with natural cheese, and anything else you desire. A short trip to the oven and violà! Not only is this kind of homemade snack less costly, it beats the cola and commercial pizza for skin health.

Sherry: What about ice cream?

Kamens: Some ice cream may be okay. Others contain replacer ingredients such as plastic cream or super-heated condensed milk. Ice cream is another product listed as "standard." The carton does not reveal the 60-odd chemicals it might contain. Beatrice Trum Hunter says:

> Ice cream is often salted. It may be homogenized. Chocolate flavor could mask spoiled flavors of other ingredients. Cheap thick-

TABLE 28
DON'T SCREAM FOR ICE CREAM
(OR: YOU'LL SCREAM WHEN YOU SEE WHAT'S IN IT)

Homemade Old-Fashioned Vanilla Ice Cream
Ingredients:
   Milk, eggs, honey, vanilla, arrowroot.

Commercial Ice Cream
Ingredients:
Note—ice cream is an FDA "Standard" product. All the ingredients contained in an ice cream package do not have to be listed on the label.

1) Can contain any number of 13 different kinds of sugar.
2) Milk can be evaporated or concentrated or sweetened or condensed or skim or dried or superheated or nonfat dry or crystallized and treated with calcium hydroxide and disodium phosphate.
3) Flavors can be artificial, coffee, tea; may contain disodium phosphate or sodium citrate.
4) Fruit can be dried, frozen, canned, whole, shredded, comminuted; it may be sweetened, thickened with pectin, or other ingredients such as agar-agar, algin, calcium sulfate, gelatin, gum acacia, guar seed gum, gum tragacanth, carrageenan, furcelleran, lecithin, psyllium seed husk and sodium carboxymethylcellulose.
5) Other ingredients: mono- and diglycerides, polysorbate 65, polysorbate 80, propylene glycol alginate, microcrystalline cellulose, dioctyl sodium sulfosuccinate, sodium citrate, disodium phosphate, tetrasodium pyrophosphate, sodium hexametaphosphate, calcium oxide, magnesium oxide, calcium hydroxide, magnesium hydroxide, calcium carbonate, magnesium carbonate.

What does commercial ice cream really contain? Even this list is incomplete. Recipes are trade secrets, Your guess is as good as ours.

From Code of Federal Regulations, FDA, #21—1977, part 100–199, pp. 174–76.

eners, beaten into the ice cream mixture to increase volume allow the ice cream to remain in an unmelted state after serving, and the gelatin or gum used for this purpose may favor germ growth in a mixture that is already a dangerous culture medium for bacteria.[118]

Dr. Ross Hume Hall, professor of biochemistry at McMaster University in Canada, is eloquent in his passionate plea for better food choices for children:

> Childhood is that time in life when the society's culture is passed on. A child's diet not only nourishes a growing body, it imprints a technical way of life, an attitude towards food and an attitude towards the functioning of one's own body. The way one approaches nourishment is learned. Young children are completely open. Recall that babies and toddlers, if given a chance, willingly consume household detergent and cigarette butts. Many tastes are acquired and it is up to the parents to provide the learning opportunities. Preference for Hostess Twinkies, Captain Crunch and catsup is not coded in human genes; neither is a preference for fresh vegetables, whole meats and whole grains. What is built into our genes, however, is an obligatory requirement for a style of nourishment that can be provided only by fresh and whole foods.
>   We know that such a diet works because our ancestors lived well on it. We are less certain of the contemporary diet of highly processed food that has come into vogue and revolutionized eating habits over the last 25 years. It has not been tested except that the population as a whole constitutes one large experiment. All evidence points to the conclusion that it is in fact a nutritionally disadvantaged diet. [It helps to have an] understanding of both the contemporary food system and the exacting requirements of your cells. The objective is to be able to sift through the food system using it to your own advantage.[119]

In conclusion, we suggest you refer to "new age" cookbooks, the kind that teach you how to make a carrot-nut cake with a nut-butter icing, a date-and-nut cupcake, or a zucchini cake.

John: A zucchini cake? Who ever heard of a *vegetable* cake?

Kamens: The name may be a turn-off to you, John, but a zucchini loaf is a "bonne bouche." You must remember that what is *familiar* sounds good. As new foods became part of your experience, you will be more at home with them.

Nutrition involves relationships between life and food. *What you eat every day of your life affects the length and quality of your entire life.* And each day, good food means more energy and better attitudes. Before the days of recorded history, people had no knowledge of nutrition as you know it today. But they didn't have to choose between an apple and a candy bar. *You* have a choice.

O! That deceit should dwell in such a gorgeous palace.
—Shakespeare, *Romeo and Juliet*, Act III
Scene 2, Line 83

Chapter 4

MAINTAINING OPTIMUM HEALTH

. . . for health is the second blessing that we mortals are capable of—a blessing that money can't buy.
—Izaak Walton, *The Compleat Angler*, Part 1,
Chapter VIII

Very few people know how to make a car. Most of us depend on General Motors. Very few people are self-sufficient when it comes to producing their own food. We depend on the supermarket. For a long time we felt assured that government controls and consumer protection were synonymous. However, there is a growing awareness that life should be less threatening than it is. It would be comforting if there were federal regulations for our safety, both in automobile manufacture and in food processing, but a number of federal regulations leave something to be desired. This is especially true when we examine the foodways of this country.

Good health flows from good nourishment, not from misconceptions. Nourishment is not vitamin A or vitamin C or calcium. Nourishment cannot be split into parts. You do not eat a single vitamin or mineral. *You do eat a carrot, or an orange, or a leafy green.* Just as every human being is an integral part of a whole, so nourishment is a *gestalt*—a totality, and only its completeness can create well-being. Once we chip, chop, divide, and attempt to reassemble bits and pieces, we lose that integrity, and with it some good health.

As we learn about the complexities of the human being, we are missing the point that the principles of health are so simple. We overlook the "helpfulness" of nature's normal elements. Some of you may remember your mothers saying, "Hurry up and eat your spinach before the doctor changes his mind about it." The confusion of parents trying to determine which foods were nourishing and which were not stemmed from the quandary of the professionals.

Let's talk about health—optimal health for children as derived from *whole natural foods*—foods that rate *ten.*

Infancy

BREASTFEEDING

Brain cells continue to develop until a baby is about six months old. If an infant is malnourished during this period, no amount of make-up nutrition at a later date will be of help. That child is stuck with a limited *number* of brain cells. If a child is malnourished after the brain cells have formed (after six months of age), the *size* (but not the quantity) of the brain cells will be affected. The brain cells actually decrease in size as a result of improper nourishment. However, the brain regains its potential size if adequate food is supplied.[1]

There is one other fact that is most commanding: When test animals are supernourished *while the brain cells are forming, the result is an increase in cells above the average quantity.*[2]

Armed with this knowledge, you obviously want your infant to be fed food of noble quality. Which food is the most exalted? Mother's milk! As technology advances we have better methods of analysis. But these only serve to reinforce the wisdom of the ages. The more we take apart, the more we respect nature.

No wonder breastfeeding is enjoying a dramatic resurgence! In its majesty, it takes care of so many problems. If a child cannot breastfeed, doctors are prescribing special formulas—but not cow's milk, the prescription of days gone by. In addition to the disadvantages of cow's milk which we have already noted, consider these facts:

☆ Cow's milk fails to provide the type of polysaccharides that feed the special protective bacteria which stand guard against enemy bacteria.[3]

☆ The calf has a tiny brain and a limited nervous system. Since its growth priority is muscle mass and bone, cow's milk furnishes a correspondingly high level of protein (3½ times the amount found in human milk).[4]

☆ Cow's milk is lower in lactose, iron, ascorbic acid, nicotinic acid, and vitamin D ... the differences between the two milks are much more subtle and diverse than previously suspected.[5, 6]

☆ The most common allergies in infants and young children are caused by cow's milk globulins.[7]

☆ The use of milk from other animals as a human food dates from comparatively recent times. The widespread use of cow's milk in infant feeding has only been made possible by the canning industry.[8]

This book is about nutrition for children. However, if you are breastfeeding, *your* nutrition will be reflected in your baby's health—despite the fact that many breast-milk nutrients are automatically regulated.

Isn't it fascinating that breastfed infants of healthy mothers have similar weight gains throughout the world until the babies are about six months of age?[9] However, there are subtle differences in quality, and these are dependent on what *you* eat. An excellent guide is the food framework and recipe section of our book, *The Kamen Plan for Total Nutrition During Pregnancy.*[10] There is great benefit derived during *lactation* by following the tenets set for good nutrition during *gestation.* Breast milk is best for the healthy infants of well-nourished women.[11]

HOW LONG SHOULD YOU BREASTFEED?

The following renowned pediatricians comment:

☆ Dr. Emory Thurston: "The mother who is truly concerned for the present and future welfare of her child will breastfeed for at least six months. A year or more is better."[12]

☆ Dr. Alvin Eden: "For those few mothers who are still breastfeeding [when the child is 18 months to two years old], there is no reason to stop. If both you and your baby are still enjoying the breastfeeding experience, then by all means continue it. You will find that your child will usually 'tell' you one way or another when [he or] she has finally had enough of breastfeeding."[13]

☆ Dr. Lendon Smith: "Separation fear or anxiety is common and is to be expected at about eight to twelve months of age. . . . Because this is a mild and short-lived problem in breast-fed babies, it seems wise to nurse a baby well into and after the months when the condition is at its peak. Try to nurse beyond one year of age."[14]

☆ Professor Derrick B. Jelliffe: "In traditional societies, including the Western world until the present century, breastfeeding was usually continued for two to three years or more."[15]

☆ Dr. C. T. Smith Clinical Nutrition: "The enzyme *ptyalin*, present in saliva, plays an important role in the digestion of starches. The power of this enzyme to perform its function is not fully developed until one year of age. It remains at optimum peak from about the first birthday until old age. For this reason, breastfeeding is essential for at least one year."[16]

NUTRIENT SUPPLEMENTATION FOR THE BREASTFED BABY

Given the biological adaptation that has occurred over hundreds of millennia, one wonders if nutrient supplements are necessary for an infant who is being breastfed by a well-fed mother. Some argue that at best, mothers today cannot be as well-fed as their ancestors because of the defects in our foodways system, pollution, environmental contaminants, and so on.

Dr. Archie Kalokerinos recommends coating the breast nipple with ascorbic acid powder just before feeding. One takes notice of Dr. Kalokerinos' recommendations based on his excellent record as medical advisor to thousands of healthy children (among whom he has totally eliminated sudden infant crib death, along with other serious but less fatal maladies). The doctor also points out that because humans do not have the ability to produce vitamin C (as most other animals do), supplementation is recommended to prevent scurvy.[17]

Iron supplements are usually added to formulas that are based on cow's milk or soy protein. The infant who is breastfed to the exclusion of all other foods does not require iron supplements. If other foods are added to the nursing child between four and six months, there is an interference of iron absorption.[18] In general, there has been a decrease in the quantity of iron supplied to infants in recent years.[19]

Despite the fact that rickets has reappeared in this country, administering vitamin D as a supplement to breastfed babies is not generally suggested. The basic cause of rickets is deprivation of sunlight. Vitamin D supplementation *may* be necessary if mother and baby cannot get enough sunlight. Prepared formulas usually contain 300 to 400 International Units of vitamin D. A similar amount is recommended for the nursing babies if they are deprived of sunlight.[20]

FORMULA FEEDING

Standards for infant formula have been published by the Committee on Nutrition of The American Academy of Pediatrics. These standards, set in 1976, have been recognized as the best possible estimate of nutritional needs of infants.[21] As we learn more, the formula will continue to improve. It is certainly a product of greater superiority than the condensed milk formulas that were probably fed to you or your parents.

Babies have their own inimitable way of saying "I've had enough." When this happens, respect the signal even though the bottle is not empty. When infants are allowed to feed on demand, they are able to regulate their energy intake with the utmost efficiency. An interesting study performed at the University of Iowa by Dr. Samuel J. Fomon very clearly demonstrates this: Two different groups of infants were fed formulas which varied in caloric content. The infants adjusted the volume of their intake so that each baby consumed the same number of calories.[22]

Infants fed formulas weigh significantly more than those infants fed breast milk and supplemental food. Part of the reason is the push to get the baby to make a clean sweep of the bottle's contents. We used to think it was "cute" when a baby's thighs were so roly-poly, a jewel thief could smuggle gems in the folds. We know better now.

One additional caveat for formula-feeding parents: Don't drop the bottle in your baby's mouth. When a baby sucks himself or herself to sleep, emerging teeth are exposed to high levels of carbohydrates—a condition conducive to dental caries development.

Since many formulas have nutrient supplements, it is best to check with your doctor about additional quantities.

ADDING OTHER FOODS

As the first year progresses, the baby's nutrient needs increase because of the rapid growth taking place. A well-fed mother can still supply about three-fourths of the major nutrient needs of her child. But that's not sufficient to meet *all* the needs.[23] It's time for the kitchen to lose its spic-and-span look, and perhaps for the dog to have additional bounty to clear from the floor: Your baby is ready for table foods.

The following suggestions should prove helpful:

☆ Dr. Robert Jackson of the University of Missouri School of Medicine: "Thriving infants should receive limited and selected amounts of solid foods after about the first six months of postnatal life. A few teaspoonsful of mashed ripe banana is suitable for an infant's early solid food. An egg yolk can be fed with the banana to provide a supplement rich in iron. Well-cooked and finely sieved legumes (peas and beans) may be used in lieu of egg yolk. After six months, it is desirable to include limited amounts of cooked cereals, sieved vegetables and fruits to provide variety in flavor and texture as well as other essential nutrients. The major source of calories, however, should continue to come from human milk until the infant is about twelve months of age."[24]

☆ Dr. J. Michael Gurney, Director of the Caribbean Food and Nutrition Institute: "The problem of weaning has been a concern of humankind since the development of our species. . . . The time when the child is becoming accustomed to the family food is fraught with danger. The use of milk from other animals as a human food dates from comparatively recent times. . . . Cow's milk is a good food but not essential for young children. . . . The ideal weaning foods are energy-dense and contain nutrients in proportion. . . . They are digestible. This implies semi-soft foods at first, becoming of a more varied and demanding texture as the child develops teeth and as his alimentary tract develops. . . . The young child's stomach is small and is growing rapidly. Therefore, feedings are required more often than for the rest of the family."[25]

BABY FOODS

In 1977, baby food sales began to plummet. The companies took action by eliminating salt and reducing sugar. But the salt and sugar issues were not the only causes for falling sales. Parents have begun to realize that with simple devices such as baby food grinders they could control the ingredients and also save money.[26]

Are you fully aware that when a can or a jar is prepared for the market, it is *heated*—a process necessary to render even a modicum of shelf life to the product? If the nutrient losses incurred in the manufacture of these foods were stated on the label, this would deter parents from purchasing them. Such labeling is virtually impossible anyway, because the nutrient losses are continuous. The longer the jars or cans sit around, the greater the losses. Temperature changes cause further losses. Who wants to feed inferior food to babies?

In the early 1970's, monosodium glutamate, a taste enchancer, was removed from baby foods. However, another palate-pleaser took its place: hydrolyzed vegetable protein, which is about 40 percent monosodium glutamate by weight![27] (The fact that hydrolyzed vegetable protein contains monosodium glutamate is not stated on the label.)

One more word of warning: Honey sometimes contains bacteria that can produce botulinal toxin once it is in the intestine of children under one year of age. This is a poison that can cause intestinal disease and sometimes respiratory failure. The American Medical Association has published a press release advising consumers against feeding honey to babies under one year of age.[28] Honey also introduces the sweet taste to babies—and we all know where that leads.

SKIM MILK: YES OR NO?

According to Dr. Fima Lifshitz and Marjorie Marks-Katz, both of the Pediatrics Department of North Shore University Hospital, Manhasset, New York, the concept that skim milk is best for babies is a myth. They say:

> It has been the fashion of late for some pediatricians to prescribe skim or low fat milk for infants who are gaining weight too rapidly and/or to avoid obesity. This is a questionable practice. When low fat milk feedings are given, the result is a dietary intake with excessively high levels of carbohydrates, protein, sodium, potassium, and chloride. This places undue stress on the baby's kidneys and requires additional water to remove the excess solute load. Furthermore, since fat is known to increase the

satiety value of the diet, low fat feedings often result in increased hunger and thus in increased food intake. The result may be that the babies end up ingesting more calories than previously taken with a regular milk.

According to the standards set by the Committee on Nutrition of the American Academy of Pediatrics, low fat milks are also deficient in vitamins C, and E, and in iron.

... Most importantly, the low fat milks lack essential fatty acids such as linoleic acid which are vital for proper infant growth and central nervous system development. Growth and central nervous system development certainly must take priority over any attempt to avoid obesity.

It is well established that breast feeding is the optimal nutrition for infants. If this is not possible, a suitable infant formula containing comparable amounts of carbohydrate, protein and fat may be substituted. If the pediatrician deems it necessary to modify the infant's diet to treat or prevent obesity, calories should not be cut by using low fat milk. Instead, the following strategies should be used:

1. Limit the amount of breast milk or formula given at feedings to just the quantity needed for proper growth.

2. Eliminate unnecessary sources of sucrose in the baby's diet, like added sugar to cereal or beverages.

3. Delay the introduction of solid foods until the baby needs it. This is usually around 6 months of age when milk formulas or breast feedings cannot provide all the essential nutrients for the baby's growth.

It's difficult to understand the persistence of doctors and nutrition counselors in their recommendations of skim milk.

SUMMARY

Well-fed mothers produce breast milk, which produces well-fed children. Cow's milk should not be fed to infants. Supplemental foods may be added after six months. Skim milk is not recommended.

In Europe, children are often weaned from the breast to yogurt. Introducing healthful foods at an early age will establish habits for a lifetime. Take advantage of your captive audience.

Growing Up

Prior to presenting *The Peanut Butter Caper,* a filmstrip in story form designed for the nutrition education of young children, we attempted to provoke participation from the twenty kindergarten children and twelve parents present at a nutrition education class. We asked, "How many of you have ever made your own peanut butter?" We addressed the question to both children and parents, and were puzzled when every child's hand went up, but not a single adult arm was raised. We repeated the question, this time directing confused glances toward the parents. Again, the same response. Now the parents were as bewildered as we were. They did not seem to know when or how their children had made peanut butter, since surely this was not in the realm of *their* culinary expertise.

We pointed to the nearest five-year-old, and asked, "How do *you* make peanut butter?" The answer came quickly: "I put the spoon in the jar, and put it on the bread. I do it myself. I make the peanut butter myself." The children all nodded in agreement, the parents laughed, and we pondered the lesson just learned: One must be keenly aware of the end products of today's foodways, and of the limits that supermarket chow imposes on a child's knowledge of what food really is. Food comes in a package. The intermediate steps of its production and consumption have diminished sharply. The ultimate is *convenience* food. The food is so convenient, that a child no longer knows that peanut butter comes from peanuts.

One mother interjected with this comment and story: She said she was relieved that other children were as confused as her own child. They had just returned from a vacation on a farm. During their stay, the child was not drinking milk. After a few days, she asked, "Gordon, what's the matter? Why aren't you drinking your milk? You usually drink several glasses a day." "Oh," said Gordon, "that was the good milk we get in the supermarket in bottles. Here it just comes from cows." What with television and books, this mother was disappointed that her child did not make the connection. Although Gordon may have been intellectually aware, his limited real-life experiences in a world of convenience foods got in the way of the cow-milk-bottle association.

o   o   o

A heartening report from College Park, Maryland, where an extensive test was conducted, concluded that *conditioning* can lead to acceptance of nutritious foods traditionally assumed to be anathema to youthful diners. The report reminisces about the hero Popeye, the comic-strip character who performed incredible feats after a mouthful or two of spinach. Before Popeye's popularity, spinach was disliked by most children. But spinach ranked second among the vegetable choices after Popeye's fame, despite the fact that it was not considered a palatable food.[29]

Nourishing the School-Age Child

You want to impart *concepts,* not *fear.* Five-year-old Danielle woke up in the middle of the night, dripping with perspiration, crying, "I ate all that junk at the party, and now I'll get sick." You can achieve a happy medium by teaching the elegance of the human body. One simple example is this: "You go into a room that is very hot or very cold, but your body remains at ninety-eight point six degrees. Your body is a great computer, and nature tends to the normal. Your computer will work, provided it is not stressed excessively. Sugar and salt and junk foods are stressors *if they become the mainstay of the diet.* When indiscretion is occasional, your body's calculator will make the adjustment.

One parent we know is troubled because her daughter is always sick in spite of the fact that she feeds her child a most superior diet. The child's playmates apparently are doing very well, and their mothers report that just a few minor changes improved their health status considerably. Everyone is an individual. Some children are exquisitely sensitive, and can only avoid illness on very pure regimens—the kind we refer to as "heroic."

The requirement is clear: Growing children must be well-nourished if they are to realize their full physical and mental potential.

A study of 700 fourth-graders conducted by the education department in Atlanta, Georgia, found that students who achieve higher scholastic levels have significantly better diets than children who are poorer students. The study shows that pupils with higher scholastic scores are more likely to eat adequate breakfasts. Higher scholastic achievement was related to adequate caloric intake, a balanced diet, and fewer empty-calorie foods.[30] Hopefully, the suggestions presented in other chapters of this book will also be helpful in bringing about changes for grade-school children.

Don't feel defeated when things get out of control. The cheating incidents will occur with less frequency as the whole family learns. When the body's blood-sugar level drops, the part of the brain that deals with self-control and conscience is altered. That's why so many people say, "Once I eat a piece of fudge, that's it." Or the alcoholic is doomed after one drink. There are biophysical changes taking place which render will power inoperative.

Adele Davis, matriarch of the "New Nutrition" movement, suggested that you advise your children that the family will eat only good food for a week, and that next Saturday you will all indulge in the "other" stuff—all the cola and pie and cakes and candy you can choke down. After a solid week solely on healthful food, most children will get very sick consuming the garbage food. It's too much of a load when they have abstained for a week. Usually, they will heave up, get headaches, and have royal stomach pains. This is a graphic demonstration of what corrupt food can do. But don't expect this to be an absolute answer: Sometimes it works and sometimes it doesn't.[31] It is human nature to forget pain and discomfort.

The New York Institute for Child Development offers this nutrition checklist[32] for your child:

1) Is there any history of allergies in the family?
2) Is there any history of diabetes or hypoglycemia?
3) Was your child colicky as an infant?
4) Were feeding problems (such as frequent formula switching) encountered when your child was an infant?
5) Did your child have any difficulty when introduced to baby/junior/solid foods?
6) Does your child have a poor appetite?
7) Does your child crave sweets?
8) Is there any food your child craves?
9) Does your child eat fruits and vegetables infrequently?

10) Is your child unusually thirsty?
11) Is your child unusually sensitive to light, noise, or touch?
12) Does your child have many colds/sore throats/ear infections?
13) Does your child complain frequently of headaches and dizziness?
14) Does your child have frequent stomachaches, constipation, or diarrhea?
15) Is your child a bedwetter?
16) Does your child have dark circles under his/her eyes?
17) Does your child have a pasty complexion?
18) Does your child suffer from eczema?
19) Does your child have a short attention span?
20) Is your child difficult to get along with?
21) Does your child cry easily for no reason?
22) Is your child depressed?
23) Is your child sleepy during the day?
24) Does your child lack energy?
25) Does your child faint if he/she eats later than usual?

If you answer "yes" to at least five (20 percent) of these questions, your child may have a physical condition that could interfere with the learning process. This checklist is designed to indicate warning signals. Peggy Charren, of Action for Children's Television, says:

> Isn't it too bad we have to think about all this? There are enough times when you have to say "No" to your children, or try to help them figure out what's right. Now we have to fight with 400 million dollars' worth of advertising money. As a concerned parent, you have to hang around the TV when the children are the viewers, and say, "No."

The Healthy Adolescent

When our daughter was thirteen, she took strong exception to the fact that we read her horoscope in the daily paper. She felt it was an invasion of her privacy. Adolescence is a time of change, of strong emotions and of departure from established norms. But it is also a time of rapidly increasing nutritional needs.[33] Your teenager will rebel against restraints and guidance. If you are just entering the food-change business, the difficulties may be magnified. However, despite the broad reach for independence, there is a tendency among young-sters to place responsibility for improper food habits and meals on their parents.[34] This may be the open door through which they can be reached.

At this age the children begin to select their own meals or food items outside the home and school. Even though penny candy is a quarter or more, the young teenager often finds ready cash for these purchases. The most popular foods are not conducive to healthful eat-ing. It is the nature of the adolescent to go on periodic food fasts, get involved in slimming programs, or skip meals and develop irregular eating habits.[35] Girls, beginning at age thirteen, consume far less ade-quate diets than previously.[36] The break comes at age ten. Even sixth-grade diets begin to decline. (And malnutrition during *any* stage of childhood impairs intellectual growth.)

Despite our plentiful supply of food, the adolescent population in this country is significantly deficient in iron, calcium, vitamin A, vita-min C, and zinc. Iron-deficiency anemia is a major problem because it is difficult to get sufficient iron intake from a "normal" diet, let alone from the imbalanced teenage diet.[37] For these reasons it is of para-mount importance that any meals consumed at home are of superior quality.

Diets should permit individual options and variety. Discuss food selections with your children. There are enough easy food alternatives to indulge everyone's fancy. Your children have a right to a certain amount of independence in food choices, provided the foods are healthful. At the risk of repetition, here again are a few easy tenets for the neophyte family:

☆ Luscious fruit! There is hardly a place where nature has bestowed her gift with a more liberal hand. Fruit exudes a savoriness that creeps gently on one's senses. Take advantage! Keep fruit bowls within easy reach.

You can play a trump card by adding green and red peppers, scrubbed carrots and raw broccoli sprigs to the "fruit of the gods," as Aeschylus called it. If you slice the fruits and vegetables, you'll guar-antee scoring points: Bits and pieces encourage consumption.

☆ Whole grains provide protective nutrients. Slowly replace the depleted varieties.

☆ Nuts in the shell, with nutcrackers at the ready, should compete with the fruit and vegetable bowls. Just set them out. They will disappear at increasingly escalating rates.

☆ Watch your own eating habits. Serving as better role models for your children is most effective.

OBESITY PROBLEMS IN ADOLESCENCE

For several Sundays in a row, the boxes of whole-wheat buns that we reserved for brunch had been pilfered. Sometimes one bun, sometimes two or three were missing. It was obvious that our teenage son was the thief. (We were about to learn a lesson about the unreliability of circumstantial evidence.) We talked to our son about his "hollow leg," and suggested other foods he could eat. We begged him to save the buns for our traditional Sunday feast, making it very clear that we did not appreciate the sneaky maneuvers he used to satisfy his insatiable appetite. Our son steadfastly denied that he was the culprit.

We were so distressed, we considered outside help for him. Finally, the truth surfaced when we returned home earlier than usual one day, and caught a twelve-year-old neighbor in our kitchen. Jane was overweight. Her parents had placed her on a stringent diet!

Dr. Anders Häger studied the obese adolescent for ten years at the outpatient obesity clinic, department of pediatrics, University of Linköping in Sweden. Here are some of his findings:

☆ As many as 50 percent of school girls have made attempts at dieting. This is the disastrous effect of a society that idolizes the virtually anorectic weight levels in popular women's magazines.

☆ Obese adolescents are extremely inactive. This may explain why the overweight teenager consumes fewer calories than normal weight controls, yet is eating more than is needed for their scanty muscular work.

☆ A prerequisite [for treatment] is a well-motivated patient. Coercion from parents is counterproductive.

☆ Total fasting means intolerable psychological stress for a growing teenager. It can result in a decrease of lean body mass and arrested height development.

☆ Treatment should start as soon as possible in an attempt to slow down the continuous division of fat cells.

☆ In late adolescence, a slow weight loss over a period of months–years is recommended.

☆ Eighty percent of obesity in childhood and adolescence persists into adulthood in spite of treatment. [Lifestle changes in eating habits and exercise ventures can change these statistics.][38]

Dr. Fima Lifshitz and Marjorie Marks-Katz have prepared a statement especially for this book. They present a strong case against weight loss during growing years:

> Obese children represent a very special problem. Unlike obese adults, they should not be treated with a weight loss diet. Caloric restriction great enough to produce a weight loss will result in a negative nitrogen balance and this will interfere with the child's growth. In adults, of course, growth is no longer a concern. Studies have shown an inverse relationship between the rate of weight loss and rate of gain in height over a period of six months or longer. Children strictly adhering to their diets have been shown to grow less than at their predicted rate or even not grow at all. The needs of all essential nutrients increase with growth and children severely restricted in their caloric intake fail to receive adequate amounts of many vitamins and minerals.
>
> Therefore, in treatment of obese children, the goal should be weight *maintenance*, rather than weight *loss*. Eventually, as these children grow, their heights will reach appropriate levels for their weights and will equalize. They will literally "outgrow their fat." In some specific conditions, under proper medical and nutritional supervision, an attempt to lose weight slowly may be made without jeopardizing growth.

The Young Adult

"Habit with him was all the test of truth, it might be right. I've done it since my youth."[39] These lines from William Shakespeare emphasize the importance of life-long practices. If you have raised your children with good nutrition regimens, you will be rewarded when they are adults. However, don't dismay when they return for their first college break looking as ghastly as the photos on their driver's license. Although they may wander the beaten path (particularly the first year away from home), they do return—especially if they've had a solid background.

But suppose you are a tenderfoot in this nutrition game? Then you and your adult children can learn together. One trick we have used to "brainwash" works very well. We buy one or two inexpensive paperback books and cut them up into two- or three-line strips. Typical:

☆ A study conducted at Cleveland's University Hospital shows that aspirin compromises the infection-fighting ability of the white blood cells.[40]

☆ Fiber in cereals is much more effective than fiber in either fruit or green vegetables in maintaining normal intestinal behavior and content.[41]

☆ Dermatologists report that vitamin B_6 alleviates "flares" of acne before menstrual periods.[42]

☆ An increase in consumption of complex carbohydrates is likely to ease the problem of weight control.[43]

☆ The overconsumption of fat, sugar, salt, and alcohol has been related to the ten leading causes of death.[44]

☆ Refined sugar not only fails to provide nutrients, but it actually robs your system of nutrients vitally needed elsewhere. The chemical systems that mobilize to metabolize sugar have to take ingredients from somewhere.[45]

☆ Nutritional status (including that of ascorbic acid) may be a critical factor in explaining why some people are susceptible to environmentally-induced diseases while others are not.[46]

☆ There is evidence suggesting a connection between dietary fat and cancer of the breast and colon.[47]

We stuff these missives into letters, into packets of vitamin supplements, into college "care" packages. We send them along with the college tuition, with reminders to call Grandma on her birthday. When the children are at home, we slip them under the napkins at the dinner table. Since the messages are brief, no one really seems to mind, even though there is a great pretense of annoyance. They not only read the words of wisdom, but share them with their friends. When our daughter was traveling, and we curtailed the brainwashing for awhile, she actually asked for the process to be continued. "You're neglecting me," she complained, "I haven't received any propaganda lately."

Our children developed reputations for being "in the know" about nutrition, and it boosted egos to have classmates ask questions they could answer with ease. Reaching the status of "master" of nutrition took time. We recall an experience our younger son had in his freshman year at college. He and his new friends were "rapping" about parent hangups. One young man said, "My parents will not discuss sex. They just don't want to hear about it." Another said, "Drugs are a forbidden subject in my home." After commiserating with each other about parents who vetoed discussions on such topics as smoking, unkempt dress, the gay scene, etc., one of the boys turned to Michael who had been quiet, and asked, "How about your parents, Mike? What's their beef?" "Well," responded Michael with honesty, "My parents get upset if I tell them I ate a chocolate bar." His classmates laughed and said, "Ah, come on, Mike—stop fooling around." Michael saw no point in convincing them that he was serious.

Getting Nutrients from Food

Everyone likes to deal in black and white. Is it or isn't it? What exactly should we do? What is the formula? But again, there are no easy answers to complex problems. With the exception of infancy, we have not outlined an optimal diet for stages of growth. We know that you know which foods are the most damaging. But it's also true that no one knows precisely what *the* optimal diet is. Dr. Mark Hegsted says:

> The fact that we do not know the optimal solution cannot and does not prevent us from using whatever relevant evidence is available to make the best judgment possible. If we wait until we know everything we need to know, we will wait forever. The issue is not the definition of an optimal diet—the issue is whether or not current dietary practice can be improved. . . . The time to start is now.[48]

And given the available knowledge, how effective is it when such strong forces are pulling in opposite directions? We can tell you about the importance of the micronutrients missing in your teenager's diet. We can tell you about the importance of chromium in normalizing endocrine function—also commonly deficient in the teen diet; about the burden of toxic minerals such as lead which cause alterations in behavior; about the ratio of magnesium, calcium, and phosphorus which impact on parathyroid gland secretions and modulate bone activity, and how these balances are thrown askew when the diets are rich in processed foods and soft drinks.[49]

All the more frustrating? Remember the cartoon of "Mama" who meets an old friend? "Do you have any children?" asks Mama. "No," says her friend. Mama responds: "So what do you do for aggravation?"

Then there's the story of the aged man who met his business partner in heaven. "Sorry it took me so long to get here. I've been on health foods."

What are "health" foods? You might say they are foods that have "class," foods packed with vitamins and minerals, with oils in natural form, and with high-quality protein. These are *nutrient-dense* foods. The more of these foods in your children's diet, the better. They may not delay visits to heaven, but they should enhance *life quality*. Here's a list of a few nutrient-dense foods:

1) Sunflower seeds (in the shell, unroasted).
2) Raw vegetables (*variety* is the key here).
3) Avocados (a marvelous fruit served as a vegetable; known as "butter that grows on trees").
4) Apples and bananas (but limit quantities; no more than 3 or 4 pieces a day at the most).
5) Homemade yogurt (do not use as main course itself; accompany each meal with a small amount).
6) Sprouts (let the children take over sprouting responsibilities).
7) Homegrown buckwheat and sunflower lettuce (teach the children how to grow these greens).
8) Garlic (a superior condiment).
9) Liver and other organ meats (see recipe section).
10) Millet (millet reigns, but a variety of whole grains should be included).

11) Eggs (fabulous protein).
12) Fish (ask your fish seller for the freshest fish from the deepest ocean).

Nature has many relay systems. There are other foods that are wholesome, but these foods are the crème de la crème of the earth's bounty. The list is short because we did not want to include unfamiliar foods, or those that are hard to come by. Most probably sprouts and sunflower lettuce have not yet beaten a path to your door. The master stroke is to incorporate as many of these jewels as possible each week, bearing in mind that too much of any one good thing is not ideal either. However, better to overload on nutritious products than on fruit juices (does your child consume quantities of apple juice?), commercial cereals (are your children Fruit Loops "freaks"?), potato chips (do they munch on these when watching TV?). The key is a *variety* of nutrient-dense foods.

Nutrient Supplementation for Children

NUTRIENT INTAKE OF AMERICAN CHILDREN

Our son Paul and a classmate were on their way back from a college sailing competition, when they found themselves on a turnpike, and hungry. Howard Johnson's was the only available food source. While waiting for dinner, Paul spread a packet of vitamin supplements on the table, and slowly chewed away on the tablets. Service was *slow* even for Howard Johnson's. Before the meal was over, Paul and his friend were arrested for pill popping. (The waitress was told to delay service pending arrival of the police.) After analyzing the contents of the pills (Paul had additional packets in his car), the embarrassed narcotics detectives apologized and paid for the college students' dinner. Brewer's yeast, desiccated liver, and ascorbic acid were not listed as "dangerous drugs."

The number of people adding nutrients to meals in condensed form has increased dramatically. The statement they are making is that the food is simply not good enough. It is not supplying everything we need for good health. But this practice may cloud the fact that nutrients are best obtained from diet. Taking vitamin and mineral supplements should not in any way reduce your personal responsibility in seeking good-food knowledge for your children, and improving their diet lifestyles. A supplement is precisely what its name implies: something added to make up for a lack or deficiency. Supplements should be used when other methods fail. If it is impossible to improve the nutritional status of a child through diet—impossible to promote health par excellence—then supplements are in order. Given the defects in our foodways system, it is a rare kitchen that turns out optimal-quality foods. However, taking out fire insurance does not prevent your house from burning down.

Are you interested in how American children stack up in terms of nutrient intake? Diets of second- and sixth-grade pupils were evaluated, together with their use of vitamin and/or mineral supplements in a public school in Illinois. The results:

☆ One half of the children take multi-vitamin supplements. Only a few take additional ascorbic acid.

☆ Most of the children are not getting enough calories.

☆ All but one child meets the allowance for protein. It is predicted that rises in food prices may alter this pattern. (We hope that additional *nutrition knowledge* will shift the precedent.)

☆ Only half of the children receive enough calcium. These are the children consuming milk.

☆ Intakes of iron are low. The use of supplements containing iron increases the number achieving better iron status.

☆ The children taking supplements have higher levels of vitamin A, ascorbic acid, thiamin, riboflavin, and niacin. However, even those taking supplements fall short of meeting requirements.

☆ The sixth-grade girls receive the lowest percentage of nutrients; the second-grade boys, the highest.

☆ Only one child in this study met 100 percent of the allowances, and this without supplementation.

☆ In most cases, second-graders come closer to meeting their requirements. At that age, they are still under parental supervision to a greater degree. The boys, in general, do better than the girls. Regardless of whether or not supplements are taken, there is a wide range of intake among the children for all nutrients.[50]

Interpreting a study like this requires insight. For starters, the gauge used was the recommended dietary allowances, which many nutrition researchers find very *limiting* for optimal health. The study considered *intake*, not *utilization*. (Forget *you are what you eat*. Change that to *you are what you assimilate*.) Nor are individual differences taken into account. There are also food antagonists to consider. The child with smoking parents has serious negative effects, requiring more vitamin C and A.[51] Overconsumption of snack foods disturbs the sodium/potassium balance; the more protein in the diet, the more B_6 required; lead toxicity is influenced by calcium and iron; sugar intake depletes nutrients; use of milk products tends to reduce nutrient absorption;[52] dietary nitrate or nitrite has been found to interfere with normal vitamin A metabolism in test animals.[53]

CONFUSION OF "NORMAL" AND "AVERAGE"

For most American women, the menstrual flow lasts five days. On superior diets, the length of time decreases to three days. Since the average flow is five days, and the optimal flow is three days, what is normal? Believe it or not, you will read in many medical texts that a *five-day* flow is "normal."

The point is that we often confuse "average" and "normal." The children in the Illinois nutrient intake study were not calcium-deficient if they had milk. However, the need for calcium is increased by *phosphorus*. (Phosphorus sources are: processed and canned meats, hot dogs, ham, bacon, processed cheese, many baked products, cola and other soft drinks, instant soups and puddings.)[54] Far less phosphorus is consumed on a natural diet than on typical American fare. Is it "normal" to require milk for calcium? Or is it "average" because of the defects in our foodways system—because of our high phosphorus intake?

In addition, the fact that the recommended dietary allowances for calcium are not being met does not necessarily indicate a calcium deficiency. Even on very low intakes of calcium, the body has amazing calcium-preservation mechanisms—especially when the food consumed is *primary* food.[55]

NOTES ON NUTRIENTS

It is obvious that the diets of our children are in a very sorry state. So—do we supplement? You may attain additional perspective after reviewing these studies:

☆ A child's iron absorption can be inhibited by large intakes of chocolate, cola, and other beverages containing caffeine.[56]

☆ Zinc deficiencies are prevalent in human populations throughout the world. Poor appetite and poor growth are signs of zinc deficiency.[57]

☆ There is no significant difference in growth when children consume zinc-fortified cereal.[58] (So much for fortification and enrichment.)

☆ Since the incidence of foodstuffs rich in vitamin C is seasonal, a large proportion of the population of the temperate and cold belts is likely to suffer for part of the year from latent vitamin C deficiency and thus be exposed to the risk of discreet metabolic disorders which may endanger the state of health. . . . For civilized communities living in a polluted environment, continuously exposed to social stress and, despite low physical activity, living on a high caloric diet rich in saturated fatty acids and sucrose, with high consumption of alcohol, cigarettes and drugs, an optimum vitamin C intake spells hope for reduction of the incidence of various metabolic disorders. (This study comes from the world review of nutrition and dietetics.)[59]

☆ Additional vitamin C minimizes the effects of nitrites.[60]

☆ A diet high in fat increases phosphorus absorption and lowers calcium levels.[61]

☆ Excessive amounts of unsaturated fatty acids (these are oils found in Italian salad dressings, peanut oils, safflower oils, etc.) can produce a deficiency in vitamin E.[62]

☆ A study showed a significant association between the presence of clinical signs of vitamin B-complex deficiency and defective vision.[63]

Obviously, the nutrients are in communication with each other. They act in concert. There is rarely a solo. The mechanisms involve interconnections among the biochemical pathways.

GUIDELINES FOR SUPPLEMENTATION

If you decide that nutrient supplementation is the route for you, these are the guidelines offered by Dr. Warren Levin of the World Health Medical Group:

The pregnant and lactating mother is routinely supplemented by her obstetrician. However, there is great controversy as to whether the newborn infant and growing child should have any nutritional supplementation. Even among those who believe as I do that such supplementation is advisable, there is difference of opinion as to quantities. My specific recommendations are:

1. A complete B-complex supplement, balanced approximately according to the formulas developed by Dr. Roger Williams, with a total intake not exceeding 5 milligrams of thiamine per day.
2. A multiple chelated mineral supplement, with calcium, magnesium, copper, zinc, manganese, iron, chromium, and selenium. Other trace minerals in small amounts are acceptable.
3. A generous pinch of ascorbic acid powder should be added to baby's bottle of water. (Even nursing infants should be supplemented with pure water—in general, in the United States. This means no tap water!) By the time a child is a year old, a supplement of about an eighth of a teaspoon a day of ascorbic acid powder—equivalent to about 500 milligrams—should be routine. At age three, the dose should be one gram. Add a gram per day for every additional year up to age ten. The dose of seven grams should be maintained after age ten.
4. One teaspoon of cod-liver oil twice per week.
5. Vitamin E, 15 units for the newborn; 30 units for toddlers; 100 units for young adults.

When children grow up taking tablets, the process becomes part of everyday living and they do not have difficulty. Our boys used to have brewer's yeast races—each would hold a handful of brewer's yeast tablets and upon signal, swallow them dry. The winner (the one to down the tablets at the fastest speed) enjoyed his reward: More brewer's yeast tablets. This may sound extreme, but it's a true story.

After watching our daughter Kathi consume a handful of supplements, a young luncheon friend asked her if she rattles when she leaves the table.

We heard Warren Klaugh, founder of Shiloh Farms, start a meal with this prayer, "Thank God I have these pills. They'll give me good vibrations and become part of me."

When we interviewed Dr. Robert Cathcart, an orthopedic surgeon from San Francisco, on WMCA Radio, he related the story of a two-year-old patient who balked at taking vitamin C, essential for his well-being because of serious ailments. The child's mother said there was no way in the world her son would take the "medicine."

Dr. Cathcart showed the child a needle, and the dose of vitamins, "Which would you rather have?" he asked. The child took the "medicine" and the mother called several weeks later to report that she never had a bit of difficulty again.

A few tricks for the recalcitrant:

☆ Coat tablets with butter. They slide down more easily that away.
☆ Wrap tablets in some applesauce or mashed banana.
☆ Grind the tablets.
☆ Teach your child to chew a bit of food, and while the food is in the mouth, practice swallowing the tablet. Once you and the children master this technique, you will never need liquids or "tricks" for swallowing tablets again.

Study the labels of chewable vitamins. Many have sugar in them.

IN CONCLUSION

If a factory requires 100 trained employees to accomplish a production goal, and only 80 are present, there are two alternatives. Either everyone works harder (that's stressful), or inexperienced outside help is brought in. Either system may work, but not as smoothly as having 100 people with expertise on the job. The supplements are the "extras." If only we could get 100 percent of requirements from our food!

Fiber Facts

Have each member of your family swallow a spoonful or two of corn kernels *without chewing them.* Examine stools in the next few days. The time elapsed from ingesting the whole kernels to the time they appear in the elimination process is known as the *transit* time. As indelicate as the subject may appear, this is an excellent gauge for determining diet status.

The transit time of an African may be about 18 hours. The average American displays a transit time of 24 to 36 *or more* hours. Transit time is dependent on fiber in the diet.

Fiber is that part of the food that doesn't break down—it's the *structure* of plants. High fiber increases fecal bulk, and produces softer, more frequent stools. A decreased transit time indicates that there is less time for possible toxins to be in contact with the intestinal mucosa. Increased bulk dilutes potential carcinogens. There is also less constipation, and therefore less sraining at stool.[64]

High-fiber foods are known as complex carbohydrates: whole grains, legumes, nuts and seeds, vegetables and fruits.

Not all complex carbohydrates have the same amount of fiber. Dr. Denis Burkitt divides foods into fiber categories. The foods with the most fiber are listed first; those with the least amount of fiber are listed last:

> Whole cereal grains—wheat, rice, corn, barley, rye, buckwheat, millet
> Legumes—peas, beans, lentils
> Nuts and seeds and dried fruit
> Root vegetables—potatoes; sweet potatoes, carrots, parsnips, turnips
> Fruits and leafy vegetables—lettuce, cabbage, celery[65]

Lettuce and apples will not give your child the kind of fiber supplied by a piece of *real* whole-grain bread. It is not surprising that a recent survey of 2,000 children shows that 75 percent of them eat fewer fruits and vegetables than deemed healthful. If Dr. Burkitt set the guidelines, chances are the percentage would near the 100 mark.[66] Fiber works in a beneficial way because it is like a sponge absorbing water, keeping the stool soft and bulky.

In addition to the fact that different foods do not have uniform fiber content, distinct *types* of fiber have divergent beneficial qualities, or different biological actions. For example, although high-fiber diets in general tend to keep cholesterol levels down, oats will lower cholesterol to a greater degree than wheat. Wheat, on the other hand, will increase transit time and stool bulk more than oats.[67] (Another testimonial for variations in diet.) Pectin, the fiber found in sunflower seeds, improves glucose (sugar) tolerance.[68]

To further complicate matters, fiber alone is not the important aspect. The *form* the fiber takes is crucial. Going back to Law #1, you can surmise that fiber in its natural form will be most effective. As an example: if you consume an apple in its whole state, or an apple that has been blended, the digestion involved in each bear little resemblance, even though it is virtually the same food product.[69] The body's response to whole brown rice is far superior to that of ground brown rice, or to whole white rice. The presence of fiber is not in itself enough to offer major benefit—the fiber must be present in a form that is effective. Studies show that that form is a whole, natural form.[70]

Only four days on a wholesome high-carbohydrate diet can cause changes that have implications for the prevention of disease.[71] After a single high-fiber meal, glucose tolerance is enhanced.

Based on all this information, it is apparent that if you are going to replace fats and sugars in the diet, the use of grains makes sense. Although we hear a lot about wheat sensitivity, many clinical ecologists believe that the troubles stem from our high technology processes. Primitive methods for preparing wheat are still in use today in parts of the world. Since it is relatively simple to grind your own wheatberries, it may be a transition step you want to consider. Wheat contains more nutrients than most people realize. As processed for commercial use today, one part of the grain is used for human food, and the rest is fed to animals. Needless to say, the most nutritious part is fed to the animals.[72]

However, although wheat may be highly nutritious, the caveat of varying your children's food applies to grains as well. You may have seen articles concerning *phytates* in grains. Phytates are concentrated in the outer layers of the grain seed. Children in India who eat chapatis as the mainstay of their diets suffer from nutritional imbalances. Chapatis (pita pouches) are unleavened, and contain more phytates than the more common Western bread. It has been shown that it is not necessarily the high phytate consumption that causes disturbances, but the lack of vitamin D.[73] Nonetheless, you will see much publicity given to the fact that *white* bread contains fewer phytates because the bran is removed, and that phytates are partially destroyed in the baking and fermentation processes.[74] But then destruction of phytate may have a deleterious effect on the biological availability of iron.[75, 76] Does it all get very confusing? Even the experts don't understand. Chances are there is an interplay—one nutrient dependent on another. The solution is to *vary, vary, vary*!!!

Exercise and Sunshine

Wait! Don't Skip Pages!

DON'T IGNORE THIS SECTION. We know that exercise and sunshine aren't exactly spellbinding subjects or Hollywood-script material, but . . .

It has been said that a nine-year-old is the nearest thing to perpetual motion in human form you will ever see. Pound for pound, he or she is the world's best endurance athlete, having the greatest heart volume for weight that the child will ever have (unless champion athletics is part of the future).[77]

Is structured exercise necessary for growing children? Regardless of how active they are, yes, exercise does encourage better health. It does keep obesity at a distance, but most of all it fosters a lifetime habit that is one of the greatest gifts you can give to your children. The easiest and least expensive exercise is walking. The family that *walks* together *talks* together. Only *doing* it will convince you of the endless advantages for each member of the family. This is especially helpful for plump adolescents. Helen Gifft, Associate Professor of Human Nutrition at Cornell, and her colleagues have explained that

> . . . an overweight teenager's negative attitude toward exercise may have numerous elements. He may know that activity uses calories but may think that it has to be vigorous to be useful. He may lack proficiency in active sports and may have resorted to sedentary interest in order to protect himself from showing up poorly before his peers. It is evident that altering his attitude will be a complex task. Correcting his faulty knowledge is one part; he needs to understand that even mild regular exercise can consume

a substantial number of calories. But facts alone are not enough; at a minimum, he will need help in improving his self-confidence and guidance toward a practical, emotionally acceptable way to increase his activity.[78]

Some youngsters are more self-directed than others. For those who lack the initiative, your invitation to walk together may work. It's a rare child who refuses time offered by a parent.

For the flexible children, practicing yoga postures has a calming effect. Establish the exercise pattern early.

Ideally, the exercise program should be done outdoors. We have always known that vitamin D may be derived from both food and the sun. However, the vitamin D obtained from the sun has a more lasting effect. In one study, it was shown that children who had a seaside holiday the previous summer had a higher concentration of vitamin D in their blood than those who had not had a summer holiday in the sun. Dietary vitamin D is relatively unimportant in maintaining circulating vitamin D. There is evidence that even in winter the concentration of vitamin D in normal people is determined largely by exposure to solar radiation the previous summer.

It is also of interest to note that too much vitamin D in the diet can lead to hypercalcemia (too much calcium); but overexposure to sunlight does not. The prolonged life of vitamin D from sunlight should encourage outdoor activities.[79]

In addition to stimulating the intestinal absorption of calcium and phosphorus,[80] sunshine vitamin D reacts in a positive way with another fat-soluble vitamin: K. The tie-in of vitamins D and K is new information.[81] Chances are as we learn more, we will become even more impressed with the value of sunshine.

ARE VEGETARIAN CHILDREN HEALTHY?

It's a familiar cartoon: the man has just exited from the supermarket, bundles in hand. He is accosted by a disreputable-looking thief who points a gun at him saying, "Okay, fella—the rib steak or your life."

Economics is one springboard for the proliferation of vegetarianism. About a third become vegetarians for health reasons. Other prime motivations could be ethical, metaphysical, ecological. Most people find they are vegetarians through a slow process of integration: They have eased themselves progressively into more strict adherence. Whatever the cause, the vegetarian *child* is on the increase.

Most forms of vegetarianism are compatible with excellent growth and good health—provided the diet follows immutable Law #1 and Law #2 (see Chapter 3).[82]

The results of an interesting study (which, in fact, was prejudiced against vegetarianism) shows that vegetarian children as a group are bright. Developmental tests reveal that the children have mental ages over a year beyond their chronologic ages. The study cites the correlation between nourishment and I.Q.[83] The researchers stated their surprise at their findings.

SUMMARY

Norman Cousins describes a new trend: people are ready to take more responsibility for their health as a new consciousness. He has commented that people are becoming less inclined to regard themselves as creatures of circumstance.[84]

You've got the computer program, but it won't work unless *you* plug it in. If ideal mental and physical health for your children is your dream, remember that "in dreams begin responsibility," and this responsibility is yours.

Chapter 5

BEHAVIOR VARIATIONS

*A child should always say what's true and speak when he
is spoken to, and behave mannerly at table;* at least as
far as he is able.

—*Robert Louis Stevenson,*
A Child's Garden of Verses;
"Whole Duty of Children"

There is the story of the poor mother who had a decision to make.
Should she send her children to school under assumed names, or
should *she* use an alias when attending P.T.A. meetings?

Dr. William G. Crook, a pediatrician specializing in children's allergies, says:

> I am absolutely certain that what a child eats can make him dull,
> stupid, and hyperactive. . . . Many effective measures in relieving
> human suffering have been used by both physicians and laypeo-
> ple alike for decades and even centuries before the reasons for
> their effectiveness were scientifically explained.[1]

Dr. Crook is modest. He offers not only anecdotes but scientific insights to help us understand behavior. Let's explore this "new"
knowledge.

The Problem Children

VICTOR

As usual, Victor was disruptive. His first-grade teacher, in familiar de-
spair, said, "Victor, there are 19 children who want to learn to read. If

you want to play, you will have to leave the room." Victor stood up, faced his peers, and said, "Let's take a vote. Who wants to read with her and who wants to play with me?" Victor's charm and high I.Q. had been an enigma since the first day of school. Why couldn't Victor cooperate, just a little?

FRED

Fred was originally diagnosed as bright but immature and as developmentally delayed. The school recommended he repeat a grade and the physician said he would outgrow the problem. Fred couldn't play baseball because he had difficulty catching and hitting a ball. He was aggressive and demanding. His handwriting was almost illegible and he often copied incorrectly from the blackboard. He had frequent headaches, pains in his arms and legs and was always tired.

DEBBIE

Debbie was labeled an underachiever. She was below grade level in reading, spelling, and math and had great difficulty completing assignments. She frequently asked to be excused from gym, was withdrawn and unhappy.

JOHNNY

Johnny was diagnosed as hyperactive at age six and was placed on ritalin. Three years later the ritalin dosage had doubled. Johnny could sit still but couldn't keep up with schoolwork. He was moody, cried a lot, had frequent stomachaches, a pasty complexion, dark circles under his eyes, and wet the bed.

Victor continued to be a "behavior" problem through the grades. He attended a special class in high school; took automotive vocational training after graduation. Victor gets by on his charm, does well and is apparently adjusted to his personal shortcomings. He cannot read and has difficulty writing. His parents feel he could have become anything he chose had he mastered the three R's. Victor says, "I choose cars. I'm okay."

The parents of Fred, Debbie, and Johnny sought professional

help at the New York Institute for Child Development. It was discovered that Fred reacted adversely to sugar and had depressed mineral levels. After a very specialized program, which included diet changes, Fred had more energy and his ability to catch and throw a ball improved. His headaches and pains disappeared. After four months of treatment he even took karate lessons. His handwriting showed marked improvement. At the end of six months, he joined little league. He was a new "Fred."

Debbie was found to be anemic and had a high cholesterol count. Her diet was low in animal and vegetable protein and high in sweets. She often saw double and was slow to focus. Words blurred on the page. Debbie's success story is exciting: After four months, she received 90's and 100's on spelling tests. After eight months she scored in the 99th percentile in math, the 94th percentile in reading. She was confident, curious, and happy.

It was determined that Johnny had possible allergies coupled with a diet poor in protein and vitamins A and C. After two weeks on a rotation elimination diet (a diet in which no food is repeated in less than four days) and developmental exercise program, his bedwetting stopped. In two months, his ritalin dosage was cut in half. After six months, he had his best school term to date, had no more stomachaches and was looking forward to his first sleep-away camp experience.[2]

All of these anecdotes are success stories, even Victor's. (Victor was lucky. He had personality and enough brain power to succeed without mastering traditional skills. He also had a supportive home background.) But how many success stories are there? How many children's lives are lacking in quality because their parents did not have the direction that Fred's and Debbie's and Johnny's had?

If you don't have a Fred, Debbie, or Johnny, you probably know one. How can we create an awareness of the relationship between *environment* (including the diet) and *behavior*, and of the incredible improvements that spring from *food modifications?*

Here's one more success story. This is about a child who wound up in a psychiatric institution. The medical staff had tried everything they could think of to help Tommy, who was a severely hyperactive child. He was uncontrollable. A student nurse pursued a technique of diet innovation. It worked! Some of the diet conversions involved using butter instead of margarine, eliminating luncheon meats; and eliminating food additives and food colorings, as outlined by Dr. Ben Feingold. Ninety days after starting the diet, Tom was ready to leave the hospital. Based on Tom's success, the staff at the hospital planned to use the "Feingold" diet on all of the children in the hospital.[3]

Behavior Difficulties: Causes and Cures

There has been an illusion that just as an individual retains the same body throughout life, so must that individual have the same mind. However, the biologists have shown that the body does not maintain a constancy in development—even for *physical* attributes. The constituents of each organ, tissue, and cell are in ongoing transition. It is because of this continuous change that we have the power to alter at least some aspects of behavior.

The human brain can be likened to a complex electronic apparatus. Instead of wires, transistors and connectors, it is 85 percent water by weight, and is referred to as a "soggy computer." Connections consist of liquids dissolved in liquids, and the brain's function is largely dependent on chemicals dissolved in this fluid. Minute amounts of chemicals can lead to disruption of brain function. Lead, caffeine, alcohol, LSD, and allergenic foods can pull the strings of behavior control.

An arsenal of nutrients are critical for brain function. These include vitamin C, the B vitamins, calcium, magnesium, and others. New orthomolecular therapies (the use of natural constituents in disease treatment) attempt to change the composition of the fluid by *detoxifying* the noxious chemicals. Increased nutrients enable the soggy computer to respond normally.

Dr. Bernard S. Rimland and Gerald Larson of the Institute for Child Behavior Research in San Diego refer to the fact that anti-social behavior results from adverse biological influences. These influences include, but are not limited to:

A) Nutrition, including
   1. Excess sugar intake
   2. Ingestion of food additives

    3. Need for increased vitamins and minerals
    4. Ingestion of phosphates
    5. Food allergy effects on behavior
 B) Pollution, including
    1. Ingestion or inhalation of lead and other toxic metals
    2. Ingestion of pesticides and herbicides inadvertently added to food or water supplies
    3. Inhalation of fumes from various environmental sources
    4. Exposure to artificial light and other sources of radiant energy
    5. Medical interventions, such as prenatal estrogen and induced delivery.[4]

It is little wonder that 10 percent of the population in the United States has handicaps or defects that are present at or develop soon after birth![5]

The large number of general learning disorders and specific deficits in behavior are of great concern. Current use of terms like "hyperactivity" and "minimal brain damage" or "special learning disabilities" are expressions of the need to explain disorders on the basis of simple relationships. Whether they are simple, or whether they are complex developmental processes, nature has many orbits. Endless studies strike at the causes of behavior and intelligence modifications. Others show how the different pathways work toward improvement.

Let's explore a few of these studies.

The Sugar Connection

☆ Dr. Richard Wurtman, a neurobiologist at M.I.T., says, "Eating sugar for breakfast could have a particularly dramatic effect on brain composition and behavior. . . . Medical history is replete with examples of anecdotes which eventually become fact. There are so many stories relating to sugar, behavior and physiological changes, it seems likely that beneath the anecdote, someday we will find fact.[6]

☆ A report in the *Journal of Learning Disabilities* by the mother of a 2½-year-old states, "As little as one teaspoon of sugar will cause constant crying, irritability and tantrums. Since taking her off sugar, I feel as though someone has given me a different child."[7]

☆ Another report in the same journal: "During the elimination diet I found it was plain old sugar out of the sugar bowl that caused the severe hyperactivity, and we suffered for three days."[8]

☆ The New York Institute for Child Development says: "We do not know the mechanism by which the ingestion of sugar is affecting these children. However, our treatment, which includes a dietary regimen nutritionally adequate, low in sugar, high in protein, with frequent feedings, has proved to be effective in helping these children. We see improvement in the ability to concentrate, longer attention spans, less irritability, less useless motion. Therefore, we have to conclude that sugar, in some way, is harmful to those particular children."[9]

The Food Additive Connection

☆ *Science* reported a study that explored hyperactivity as caused by additives. The study shows that hyperactive children who typically ingest 100 or 150 milligrams of additives a day will demonstrate very marked behavior changes.[10]

☆ Dr. Doris Rapp of Buffalo, New York, studied 24 hyperactive children, selected at random. She found that 75 percent of them were made hyperactive by foods and food colors, dyes, and additives. A majority of these children also suffered from symptoms of the allergic tension-fatigue syndrome including headaches, bellyaches, leg aches, bedwetting, and stopped-up noses. Dr. Rapp confirmed her findings using double-blind techniques.[11]

☆ The antioxidants BHA and BHT, which are on the Feingold exclusion list, produce behavioral changes in test animals.[12]

The Nutrient Connection

☆ Dr. Lendon Smith explains that calcium deficiency is responsible for a lot of hyperactivity. Smith cautions that if a child has twitchy movements and craves milk, he or she is probably looking for calcium, and/or is not absorbing it. The milk allergy prevents the calcium from being absorbed.[13]

☆ The program director for nutrition at the Institute for the Study of

Mental Retardation and Related Disabilities at Ann Arbor, Michigan, reports: "... some children with developmental disabilities have ascorbic acid needs higher than the recommended allowance for the normal population.[14]

☆ From the London School of Hygiene and Tropical Medicine: "... Children who have been continuously well nourished ... created around themselves a stimulating environment by their attention-seeking, demanding, exploratory, and active behavior. This was in marked contrast to the ... child who was moderately malnourished during infancy and early childhood, and was characteristically 'well behaved'—notably quiet, timid, sad, apathetic, minimally mobile, with delayed speech and motor milestones—growing up in his own little environment of deprivation and minimal stimulation.[15]

☆ Rimland and Larson: "Damage incurred in infancy may increase the brain's need for a certain substance to a level that would not ordinarily be reached by eating a normal diet, but might be reached by using potent nutritional supplements.[16]

☆ *The Proceedings of The National Academy of Sciences* reports highly significant gains in *IQ* in a group given vitamins. The effect of the supplements not only improved *IQs*, but also physical health and growth.[17]

☆ A study done at the Naval Academy, class of 1980 by Rimland, Montor, and Afdahl, shows that students who had significantly higher grades in several subjects also had higher levels of vitamin C.[18]

The Phosphate Connection

☆ From Heidelberg, Germany, we review a report that indicates that when hyperactive children are fed phosphates for several weeks, hyperactivity will commence almost immediately. There may even be *symptoms of minimal brain damage*.[19] The phosphate problem is gaining widespread attention. Lendon Smith states that the high phosphorus content in the children's diet is responsible for the calcium deficiency.[20] Once again, here's a list of the foods containing phosphates:

Almost all processed or canned meats (hot dogs, ham, bacon)
Processed cheeses
Baked products which use phosphate baking powder (commonly used)

Cola drinks; other soft drinks
Instant soups and puddings
Toppings, seasonings[21]

The Allergy Connection

☆ In 1956, Dr. William Crook became interested in the relationship
of food allergy to chronic and sometimes ill-defined complaints when
an alert mother convinced him (against his will) that her twelve-year-
old son's headache, irritability, fatigue, and nervousness decreased
dramatically when she removed milk from his diet.[22]

☆ A report in *Annals of Allergy* shows that a survey of hyperactive
children responded to a sensitivity test and the magnitude of the response was significantly correlated with teacher's ratings of hyperactivity and inattentiveness.[23]

☆ Research quoted in *Biological Psychiatry* demonstrates in a double-blind study that allergic exposure provokes psychological symptoms.[24]

☆ According to Dr. Frederic Speer, a Kansas clinical ecologist, the
more common offending foods are:

Cow's milk
Chocolate and cola (the kola nut family)
Corn (i.e., Cracker Jacks, tortillas, Fritos, burritos)
Eggs (i.e., mayonnaise, breaded foods, noodles, icing)
Pea family [chiefly the peanut] (i.e., snap beans, dry peas, etc.)
Citrus fruits (oranges, lemons, limes, grapefuits, tangerines)
Artificial food colors (i.e., Hi-C, Tang, Kool-Aid, Popsicles, Jell-O,
    heavy antibiotic syrups, soda, etc.[25]

☆ *In questioning parents of children with behavior disorders, the parents indicated that removal of milk, wheat or sugar from the diet was
more effective than psychotherapy.*[26]

The Lead (and Other Toxic Metals) Connection

☆ *The Journal of Pediatrics:* "There was a significantly higher level
of copper in children who were reported to respond to restricted diet

compared to those children who apparently had no response. The restricted diet administered was the Feingold diet." The study shows that an elevation of blood copper concentration in hyperactive children responding to the Feingold diet, may offer a clue to one possible biochemical mode of action. The action is the consequence of chemicals added to the modern diet.[27]

☆ A comparison of dyslexic children and normal children shows a significantly higher concentration of magnesium, copper, and aluminum in the dyslexic children. The cadmium levels were so high in these children that they also exceeded the normal acceptable range. The results indicate that excessive cadmium may be implicated in this form of learning disorder.[28]

☆ *The American Journal of Psychiatry* reports a study showing that blood lead concentrations were higher in mentally retarded children for whom no cause could be found for their retardation than in those in whom a cause was highly probable.[29] (Lead leached from solder in the seams of food cans and from the plugs sealing evaporated milk cans contributes about 14 percent of total dietary lead, according to Food and Drug Administration estimates.)[30]

☆ Measuring levels of a few minerals and metals, including lead and cadmium, was a clue to pinpointing children with problems. Dr. R. O. Pihl could select the learning disabled and behaviorally disordered schoolchildren with almost 98 *percent accuracy* based on these tests![31]

☆ Boston's Children's Hospital and Harvard Medical School asked children to save their fallen teeth, not for the tooth fairy, but for an unusual experiment. The teeth were tested for lead levels. High lead levels easily matched those children who were less competent in areas of verbal performance and auditory processing. They had reduced attention spans, daydreamed more, and exhibited lower intelligence scores.[32] Alexander Schauss, who has done intensive work on the relationship between lead and behavior, points out that the levels found to affect the school children's behavior was *below* what is usually considered a *toxic* level.[33]

Once again we refer to nature's numerous pathways for accomplishing the same goal. There are many substances that help the body "chelate" or get rid of toxic metals. Research describing these substances follows:

• ⊙ •

☆ Dr. Carl Pfeiffer of The Brain Bio-Center in Princeton, N.J., says: "If toxic substances enter the body, adequate *vitamin C* often detoxifies them, rendering them harmless. Vitamin C's effectiveness has been demonstrated in correcting the toxic effects of lead, iron, copper, bromide, arsenic, benzene, and the pesticides DDT, dieldrin, and lindane.[34]

☆ John Kirschmann, Director of Nutrition Search, Inc., and author of the very well researched *Nutrition Almanac,* states: "The single most effective way to prevent lead poisoning is to include a small amount of *algin* in the daily diet. Algin is a nonnutritive substance found in Pacific kelp, which is sometimes used as a thickening agent in the preparation of various foods. It attaches itself to any lead that is present and carries it harmlessly out of the system."[35]

☆ Dr. Denis Burkitt, world-renowned surgeon, and recipient of the gold medal of the British Medical Association: "*Fiber* interacts with various poisonous substances in the feces (the name given to the content of the bowel), and prevents their absorption into the circulation of the body. In this way poisonous substances are eliminated from the body instead of being absorbed."[36]

☆ A report in the *Journal of the American Medical Association,* using test animals, indicated that adequate dietary calcium prevents accumulation of lead in body tissues by reducing absorption of ingested lead from the intestinal tract.[37]

The Pesticide and Herbicide Connection

Many of the mechanisms involved in the metal toxin influence on behavior apply to the pesticide and herbicide influence. We know, for example, that inadequate consumption of zinc may enhance the toxicity of DDT. Dietary exposure to several insecticides diminish the body's stores of vitamin A. Not only the quantity, but the *quality* of protein is essential in maintaining levels of vitamin A in the presence of pesticides. Methionine, an amino acid found lacking in legumes, is an important factor. In addition, sulfur-containing amino acids (as found in eggs) can prevent DDT-induced depletion of liver vitamin-A stores.[38]

Low levels of calcium enhance the toxicity of several chlorinated hydrocarbon insecticides.[39] Lindane, another pesticide, is excreted in great quantities when the diet is comprised of fiber, including fiber which contains pectin.[40] Individuals consuming high-fat diets may enhance their susceptibility to insecticides.[41]

The incidence of *multiple* interactive factors weave a tangled web. If herbicides and insecticides reduce nutrients, and nutrients affect behavior and intelligence, the herbicide and insecticide influence is obvious. It's a two-way street. Natural food substances diminish body burdens of these contaminants.[42]

Other Environmental Connections

Sadly, one of the most important sources of carbon monoxide is not environmental pollution in general, but personal pollution by cigarette smoking. The concentrations produced by cigarette smoke are far higher than would occur even in the most polluted atmosphere of Los Angeles.[43] In addition to carbon monoxide problems, a recent study of more than 17,000 children in England showed that the children of smokers were four months behind in reading at 7 years of age compared with children of nonsmokers. There is also clear evidence that prenatal exposure to smoking affects other aspects of behavior.[44]

We are increasingly *creating* our environment, and with it, a peck of troubles. Chemical products and byproducts of our technologically advanced society have very special implications for children because they are in the growth process. Tissues and cells that are proliferating and maturing are more sensitive to any toxin.

The Artificial Light Connection

Dr. John Ott, a photobiologist, has brought to our attention the relationship between children's behavior and malillumination. Children subjected to long hours of artificial light that cuts out some of the natural rays of "full spectrum light" respond unfavorably. Lack of natural light may be considered a nutritional deficiency. Full-spectrum fluorescent tubes are available.[45]

Needless to say, the best balanced light exposure comes from spending some time outdoors. There is a supreme benefit when you get into the family "walking-together" habit: Everyone gets that natural light on his or her face—so essential for optimal health *and behavior.*

The Drug Connection

The effects of drugs start in pregnancy. A study reported in *Science* in 1978 states:

> When babies were tested at 4 month, 8 months and 12 months of age, those whose mothers were heavily medicated during pregnancy lagged in the development of the ability to sit, stand, and move about. They were also deficient in developing inhibitor abilities, such as the ability to stop responding to redundant signals, to stop crying when comforted, and to stop responding to distracting stimuli. As they grew older, their development of language and cognitive skill lagged or was impaired.[46]

Antihistamines are a common constituent of cold remedies. Joe Graedon, in *People's Pharmacy,* describes the consequences of administering antihistamines to children: "Central nervous system stimulation [is often the result], causing insomnia, nervousness and irritability."[47]

Salicylates have been indicted as a substance responsible for hyperactivity. Some drugs cross-react with salicylates. Aspirin is a drug containing salicylates.[48] For the hyperactive child, aspirin is definitely not desirable. Another development often encountered from the ingestion of aspirin is *tinnitus*—which manifests itself with ringing in the ears (or buzzing or roaring). The child is cranky as a result of an earache. Aspirin is given to relieve symptoms, and a vicious cycle commences.[49]

Home Behavior Evaluation

How can you possibly know if your child is under stress because of physical imbalances? Isn't it possible that behavior variations may be caused by psychological pressures? Stress, regardless of cause, depletes nutrients. Symptoms may be similar: Poor school performance; erratic behavior; headaches and stomachaches; irritability and an inability to concentrate.

Dr. Jerome Vogel, of the New York Institute for Child Development, warns that stress can seriously threaten your child's physical and mental well-being. He says:

> Children under stress all have something in common: Frustration, poor self-image and a feeling of helplessness. The impact on the entire family can be devastating. Stress is part of a vicious cycle.... Prolonged stress resulting from a child's inability to cope with his [or her] environment can trigger biological imbalances such as vitamin and mineral deficiencies, abnormal response to sugar and allergic reactions. Even if a child is under external or emotional stress, the internal system is affected. If a child is failing in school or is hyperactive or overweight because of an emotionally charged home situation, his or her internal system will often correct itself once the emotional problem is cleared up. This is not true of a child who is failing or is a behavior problem because of a biological imbalance. No matter what you try to do, this child will continue to have problems until the specific biological imbalance is properly diagnosed and treated. If stress is allowed to continue unchecked, serious problems can result in later years. The stressed child going into adolescence is more likely to become involved with drugs, alcohol and juvenile delinquency. As an adult, there is greater susceptibility to heart attacks, ulcers and high blood pressure.

To help you determine the basis and extent of your child's stress, Dr. Vogel has developed *The Children's Stress Test.* The test is based on years of work with children previously diagnosed as learning disabled, hyperactive, overweight or underachieving.

PRE-SCHOOL AGE

1. Is your child afraid of heights (i.e., won't climb on Jungle Jim; doesn't like to be picked up)?

2. Is your child extremely daring?
3. Is your child easily distractible?
4. Is your child always up and down from the table during meals?
5. Is your child a discipline problem?
6. Does your child seem to "tune-out" at times?
7. Does your child find it necessary to touch everything he/she sees?
8. Does your child frequently walk into things or trip?
9. Is there inconsistency in your child's performance (i.e., one day he/she performs a task well, the next day he/she can't)?
10. Does your child have a short attention span?
11. Does your child get frequent headaches?
12. Does your child frustrate easily?
13. Does your child have difficulty keeping rhythm while dancing or clapping?
14. Is your child usually sensitive to light, noise, touch or certain clothing material?
15. Was your child a late walker?
16. Was your child a prolonged tiptoe walker?
17. Was your child's speech late or abnormal?
18. Does your child have frequent nightmares?
19. Is your child a bedwetter?
20. Does your child have uncontrollable rage reactions?
21. Does your child complain of seeing things bigger or smaller than they are?
22. Is your child always tired?
23. Is your child unable to keep up with the other children's activity levels?
24. Does your child have a poor appetite?
25. Does your child have a history of anemia of any type?
26. Is your child irritable before and/or shortly after meals?
27. Is your child easily fatigued?
28. Does your child exhibit excessive thirst?
29. Does your child crave sweets?
30. Has your child experienced excessive weight gain or loss?
31. Did your child have trouble learning to skip?
32. Does it seem that your child never pays attention to you?
33. Is your child unable to modulate his/her voice?

34. Does your child keep his/her head very close to the paper or tilt it back and forth when reading or writing?
35. Does your child have frequent stomachaches?
36. Does your child frequently go out of the lines when coloring?
37. Did your child have trouble learning how to tie and/or button and/or lace?
38. Does your child always seem to have a cold?
39. Was your child colicky?
40. Was your child an unusually cranky baby?
41. Was your child an unusually passive baby?
42. Does your child do everything to excess (i.e., laugh, cry, talk, sleep, perspire)?
43. Does your child have poor bowel or bladder control?
44. Does your child seem preoccupied with matches, fire, etc.?
45. Is your child a bully?
46. Is your child always picked on by his/her peers?
47. Is your child a loner?
48. Does your child's walking or running seem clumsy or disjointed?
49. Is your child ever purposely destructive?
50. Does your child have a history of allergies?

GRADES 1–8

1. Does your child have difficulty understanding what he/she reads?
2. Does your child avoid sports or activities that involve catching and throwing a ball?
3. Is your child very afraid of heights (i.e., won't climb on the Jungle Jim; doesn't like to be picked up)?
4. Is your child extremely daring?
5. Does your child's running seem uncoordinated or sloppy?
6. Does your child get lost frequently?
7. Is your child easily distractible?
8. Does your child confuse right from left?
9. Does your child use one hand for some things and the other hand for other things?
10. Is your child always up and down from the table during meals?

11. Is your child a discipline problem?
12. Does your child go up or down stairs one step at a time?
13. Does your child seem very bright and articulate when in conversation but cannot seem to understand what he/she reads?
14. Is your child the class clown?
15. Is your child not working up to his/her potential?
16. Does your child seem to "tune-out" at times?
17. Is your child unusually forgetful?
18. Does your child find it necessary to touch everything he/she sees?
19. Does your child frequently walk into things or trip?
20. Is there inconsistency in your child's performance (one day performs a task well, the next day can't?)
21. Does your child have a short attention span?
22. Does your child move his/her lips while reading or follow the line with his/her finger?
23. Does your child get frequent headaches?
24. Is your child ever purposely destructive?
25. Does your child frustrate easily?
26. Is your child unusually sensitive to light, noise, touch, or certain clothing material?
27. Was your child a late walker?
28. Was your child a prolonged tiptoe walker?
29. Was your child's speech late or abnormal?
30. Is your child a bedwetter?
31. Does your child have uncontrollable rage reactions?
32. Does your child complain of seeing things bigger or smaller than they are?
33. Is your child unable to keep up with the other children's activity levels?
34. Does your child have a poor appetite?
35. Does your child have a history of allergies?
36. Is your child irritable before and/or shortly after meals?
37. Does your child crave sweets?
38. Has your child experienced excessive weight loss or gain?
39. Does your child frequently go out of the lines when coloring?
40. Did your child have trouble learning how to tie and/or button and/or lace?
41. Was your child colicky?

42. Was your child an unusually cranky baby?
43. Was your child an unusually passive baby?
44. Is your child a bully?
45. Is your child always picked on by his peers?
46. Is your child a loner?
47. Does your child seek out older or younger playmates?
48. Does your child's walking or running seem clumsy or disjointed?
49. When your child reads out loud, does he/she get mixed up or lose his/her place?
50. Does your child not complete his/her homework assignments?

HIGH SCHOOL

1. Does your child avoid sports or activities that involve catching or throwing a ball? Or did he/she?
2. Does your child's walking or running seem uncoordinated or sloppy?
3. Is your child easily distractible?
4. Does your child confuse left from right?
5. Is/was your child always up and down from the table during meals?
6. Is your child a discipline problem?
7. Does your child seem very bright and articulate when in conversation but cannot seem to understand what he/she reads?
8. Is your child the class clown?
9. Is your child below grade level or not working to his/her potential?
10. Is your child unusually forgetful?
11. Does your child frequently walk into things or trip?
12. Is there inconsistency in your child's performance?
13. Does your child have a short attention span?
14. Does your child move his/her lips while reading or follow the lines with his/her fingers?
15. Does your child get frequent headaches?
16. Does your child frustrate easily?
17. Does your child have difficulty keeping rhythm while dancing or clapping?

18. Was your child a late walker?
19. Was your child a prolonged tiptoe walker?
20. Was your child's speech late or abnormal?
21. Does your child complain that words blur or move on the page?
22. Is your child always tired?
23. Does your child have a poor appetite?
24. Does your child have a history of anemia of any type?
25. Is your child irritable before and/or shortly after meals?
26. Does your child exhibit excessive thirst?
27. Does your child crave sweets?
28. Has your child experienced excessive weight gain or loss?
29. Did your child have trouble learning how to tie and/or button and/or lace?
30. Was your child colicky?
31. Was your child an unusually cranky baby?
32. Does your child do everything to excess?
33. Does/did your child have poor bowel or bladder control?
34. Is your child a bully?
35. Is your child always picked on by his/her peers?
36. Is your child a loner?
37. Does your child seek out older or younger playmates?
38. When your child reads out loud, does he/she get mixed up or lose his/her place?
39. Is your child ever purposely destructive?
40. Does your child complete his/her homework assignments on time?
41. Is your child often truant from school?
42. Does it seem your child never pays attention to you?
43. Is your child unable to modulate his/her voice?
44. Does your child keep his/her head close to the paper or tilt it back and forth when reading or writing?
45. Does your child always seem to have a cold?
46. Does your child get frequent stomachaches?
47. Does your child seem to "tune-out" at times?
48. Does your child have uncontrollable rage reactions?
49. Does your child have a history of allergies?
50. Was your child an unusually passive baby?

The Institute suggests that if you have answered "yes" to at least 10 (or 20 percent) of the questions, it may be that your child has a learning disability. This does not mean that your child is unintelligent. On the contrary, most children who suffer from learning disabilities have at least average and often above-average intelligence. It is advisable to investigate the medical, biochemical, nutritional, and functional disorders that cause hyperactivity and learning problems. Before any child can achieve full potential, the biochemical and neurological systems must function properly.

IN CONCLUSION

The hinges and corking pins, the blends and bonds, the integration of the known and as yet unlearned nutrients and their mechanisms can be mind-boggling. But the bottom line remains unchanged: include nutrient-dense food in your child's diet, and minimize any negative nutrient substances. Laws of Choice #1 and #2!

Let's remember Dr. William Crook's words, "What a child eats can make that child dull, stupid, or hyperactive." On the other hand, what a child eats can make that child bright, smart, and well-balanced.

Chapter 6

MENU FOR THE SICK AND FOR MINOR MALADIES

Who shall decide when doctors disagree?
—Alexander Pope, Moral Essays, *Epistle*
II: Line 261

"But I don't want to go to the doctor." Four-year-old Georgie was in tears. His father tried to console him. "The doctor only wants to *look* at you." "Then why don't you send him my picture?" This conversation could not have taken place a hundred years ago. In those days very few families went to the doctor, and even fewer had pictures. If a doctor happened to live in your community, chances are he would visit *you.* But you would not send for him unless Grandma's remedies failed. The number of hours or days elapsing between the time your message was received by the good doctor *and his arrival* depended on his horse, the trail, the weather, and how many requests preceded yours.

Fortunately, Grandma's use of elixirs (which her Grandma taught *her*) usually worked for most minor problems. We learn from studying ancient and traditional pharmacopoeia that most illnesses are universal. However, solutions vary—again emphasizing nature's many relay systems, not only internal, but external as well. For example, people get colds the world over. Indians drank a tea of native evergreen forest hemlock to relieve symptoms.[1] A Russian folk remedy for the same discomfort: finely grated horseradish mixed with lemon juice.[2] The Rumanians use comfrey root, while the Italians resort to garlic. Africans sniff pinches of cayenne pepper. A pint of milk and an ounce of chopped fresh ginger root are simmered in a small teakettle in Asia, and the rising vapors are swallowed. Outer Mongolians consume a cup of hot yak milk embellished with grated garlic and ghee.[3] The recovery techniques are as dissimilar as ethnic backgrounds.

Here are some more diverse traditional nostrums for sundry ailments:

Burns:
> carbolic acid, bicarbonate of soda and linseed oil
> butter
> tannic acid

Kidney troubles:
> parsley
> cornhusk silks

Bad blood:
> burdock root
> diluted lemonade
> comfrey leaves

Chilblains:
> parsnips
> alum
> cayenne and talcum powder mixture in shoes

Nerves:
> potassic tartrate of iron
> warm bath

General malaise:
> chicken soup

Some of the old afflictions have all but disappeared (diphtheria, polio, plague). Others have come to take their place. In a vintage household medicine guidebook, you'll see many of the above suggestions, but you won't find hints for dealing with baby powder aspiration, immunization reactions, methylmercury poisoning, DES-caused vaginal cancer, additive-induced hyperactivity, atomic fallout exposure, etc.

Whether the disorders can be identified with established diseases of history, or whether they are the outgrowth of late-twentieth-century technology, a few facts remain the same:

1) The state of an illness is a manifestation of the degree of health. The malnourished child is more susceptible to severe consequences of measles, developing major complications from the

disease more readily than a child who is well nourished. Malnutrition impairs the immune response.[4] Or, as outlined in Chapter
5, the nutrient-equipped body is less prone to lead toxicity.
2) Well-nourished bodies heal more rapidly.
3) Only *you* can be responsible for your own recovery. The doctor
cures no one but himself or herself.

Rising costs of medical care may cause fundamental changes. Hopefully, this will lead to an awakening of the *real* cause of illness. Even
Congress sees *prevention* as a promising "cure," and, in an attempt to
accomplish this goal, offers advice to everyone.[5] Of course we do have
to overcome difficult existing barriers which block the improvement
of dietary practices, but while we are slowly attempting to get
through the breakwaters, the children will exhibit the effects of all the
indiscretions thrust upon them: *They will get sick from time to time.*
    The chief requisite for healthy growth is nutrition. Exercise im-
proves nutritional mechanisms, and stress decreases them, but good
food is the lifeline. *It is natural to be well.* The body wants to be well.
When health breaks down, it is an expression of the body's effort to
shake off conditions and/or substances that oppose health. The body
strives toward health when any disturbance is present.
    Symptoms can be artificially suppressed with the use of drugs.
This is the way of the traditional physician. There are times we are
grateful for such knowledge. However, if you examine and question
causes each and every time your child is ill, you will be brought closer
to understanding the concept of disease and healing, and ultimately
the maintenance of good health.

Allergies

    Over two thousand years ago Lucretius said, "What is food to one
man may be fierce poison to others."[6] It is true that individual idio-
syncracies exist—each and every food probably gives someone an allergic reaction. *But countless numbers of people the world over are
sensitive to a few select foods.* Given the fact that food choices have
narrowed (don't be fooled by the 30,000 supermarket "selections")

and given that reactions to a few foods have increased, we may have to rephrase Lucretius: "What is poison to one person may indeed be poison to others." The commonly offending foods include milk, wheat, corn, chocolate, citrus fruits, nuts, and eggs.

Allergy tests are not always reliable. Many children who do not test positively for (or show signs of) milk intolerance, but who have indications of allergies, are in fact allergic to cow's milk. When these children refrain from ingestion of cow's milk, symptoms totally disappear.[7] Milk consumed by a *mother* may even affect her *baby:* When a group of breastfeeding mothers complained of having infants with colic, they were advised to go on milk-free diets. The mothers eliminated milk from their diets, and the babies' colic disappeared promptly.[8]

Dr. William Kaufman provides interesting allergy facts: food-induced allergic illnesses may occur only occasionally, or they may occur often. Usually a child reacts to those foods which he or she has eaten with great frequency or in very large amounts. *Chronic* disorders result from foods eaten daily. This is the reason that variety in food choices is recommended.

The major problem in allergy treatment, explains Dr. Kaufman, is identifying the offending food. To date, the most accurate method of accomplishing this is to eliminate the suspect food for a period of time, and then reintroduce it. The other tests are not infallible. The fact that there are no visible signs of allergy does not necessarily mean that an allergy does not exist. The manifestations of allergies may differ. They tend to be dose- and frequency-related on an individual basis. A fraction of a drop of cow's milk may cause a reaction in one child, whereas it may take a quart of milk to induce symptoms in another child.

Allergic reactions usually take 18 to 36 hours to manifest themselves, although some reactions may occur in 15 minutes. An allergic response also favors retention of salt and water for the duration of the allergy. Among the symptoms of allergy are pallor, puffiness under the eyes, and weight gain from the water retention. According to Dr. Kaufman, most children do not outgrow allergies. However, their manifestations change. The child who breaks out in hives from strawberries when young, may develop a headache when older. Allergic reactions at any age are very diverse, making it difficult for the doctor who is not familiar with food-induced allergic syndromes to recognize them as such. The most effective methods of detecting allergenic foods include analysis of a carefully taken history, a food-symptom-daily-happening diary, and an elimination diet (eliminating the offending foods and observing reactions).

Dr. Kaufman suggests that once the troublesome food is identified, eliminate the food from the diet in every form. This is not easy as your child must be emotionally prepared for a change in diet, and you must be prepared for your child's behavioral reactions to deprivation of familiar foods.[9]

Thousands of children receive allergy shots on the basis of skin tests that are incorrectly performed or erroneously interpreted, or both.[10] Milk is the most frequently allergenic food. Of 1,000 food-allergy cases examined (all ages), 680 were allergic to milk. While early milk allergy may be outgrown, there is a strong tendency for it to persist into adult life.[11] Skin tests are not dependable. A two- or three-week trial elimination of milk is the most reliable diagnostic procedure. After the elimination diet, foods should be introduced cautiously and one at a time by feeding a small portion on an empty stomach, preferably one hour before the midday meal.[12]

When an infant has cow's-milk allergy, it is recommended that the following foods be eliminated from the diet (in addition to all foods containing cow's milk) until the child is two years old: citrus fruit, chocolate, egg, nuts, peas, and fish. Many of these foods are known to have caused symptoms in children with cow's milk allergy.[13] The length of breastfeeding needed to prevent cow's-milk allergy is not known, but prolonged breastfeeding reduces the frequency of other forms of allergy, too.[14]

Allergic infants in Europe and Asia are fed yogurt prepared from fresh cow's milk or goat's milk, beaten until the curds are small. Acidophilus culture is often tolerated by milk-allergic children. This type of lactic acid food acts as a valuable antihistamine.[15]

Infants who are extremely sensitive to cow's milk may respond with severe symptoms to a diaper ointment (Diaparene Neonatal Ointment). The ointment contains casein, a milk protein. This report is brought to your attention for several reasons. It emphasizes both the intensity of a reaction to a medication applied *topically,* and the subtlety of some reactions. Had one mother not been aware of cow's-milk-allergy symptoms, she would not have been able to assist the doctors in determining the cause of her baby's almost fatal reaction. The doctor reporting this incident stresses that more than likely, if looked for, reactions of equal, lesser degree and even greater intensity may be uncovered.[16]

Milk-sensitive children should not have any of the following foods: buttermilk, chocolate milk, skim milk, light or heavy cream, sour cream, butter, sherbet, nondairy products that may have milk solids added, evaporated milk, powdered milk, puddings, bakery products made with any of these items, creamed soups, creamed sauces, gravies, all cheeses, nondairy substitutes containing *caseinate,* such as Coffeemate, Cereal Blend, Preem, Rich'ning, Cool Whip. (Caseinate is a milk protein.) Cultured products such as yogurt may be more easily tolerated. Pancakes, waffles, omelets, puddings, and creamed dishes may have milk products in them.[17, 18]

Since milk allergies are so common, you may be wondering whether or not *your* child is milk-sensitive. Common symptoms to milk intolerance: stomach and other cramps, diarrhea or loose stools, nausea and sometimes vomiting, flatulence, bloating, nasal symptoms including mucus, fatigue, eczema, asthma, behavior disturbances, colic.[19]

Wheat-sensitive children: Omit all bran products, pancakes, waffles, breads, cookies, crackers, cakes, breaded foods, pasta. The safest grains are the gluten-free grains such as brown rice, millet, and buckwheat. (Rye, barley and oats contain gluten.) Avoid fried foods. (June Roth, author of *Aerobic Nutrition,* suggests that you can create a batter made of seasoned beaten egg whites.[20])

Many rye products contain wheat, as do most of the commercial cold cereals. Since malt resembles wheat, this too should be eliminated. Flour *mixtures* often contain wheat. Other wheat-containing items are: bouillon cubes, chocolate candy, cooked mixed meat dishes, fats used for frying foods rolled in flour, fish rolled in flour, fowl rolled in flour, ice cream cones, most cooked sausages, thickenings in ice cream, anything breaded, zwieback, and anything with gluten (which is a wheat protein).[21]

Egg-sensitive children should avoid mayonnaise, creamy salad dressings, meatloaf, pancakes, waffles, malted cocoa drinks, cake mixes, breads, breaded foods, ice cream, pasta, marshmallow. Dried egg is a frequent addition to processed foods.[22]

These products may contain corn, and should be avoided by *corn-sensitive children:* Bacon, baking powders, batters for frying, breads and pastries, candy, carbonated beverages, processed cereals, catsups, chewing gums, jams and jellies, lemonade, noodles, peanut butter, pork and beans, puddings, sherbets, vitamins, popcorn, corn oil, corn syrup, hominy grits, and cornbread.

The post office is the largest customer for dextrin: It's used as glue on stamps and envelopes. Dextrin is a corn derivative.[23, 24]

Chocolate-sensitive children should not have chocolate, cocoa and cola, or cola-flavored foods. This includes chocolate candy, cakes, cookies, pies, and chocolate milk. Low-calorie cola drinks need to be avoided. Most cola drinks are made from cola nuts, which are related to cocoa beans. Carob, however, is acceptable.[25]

Dr. William Holub, Professor of Nutrition and Biochemistry at C. W. Post College in New York, points out that allergy results from an inadequate nutritional support causing defective internal detoxification. He concludes that treatment of allergy requires far more than the identification and isolation of the allergen. It requires a program of dietary regulation and food supplementation to ensure adequate detoxification.[26]

Acne

Skin disorder? Eat raw grated potato. Blemished skin? Celery juice. Or maybe spinach and carrot juice. These are old gypsy remedies. Interesting, especially the carrot juice suggestion—in light of recent findings concerning vitamin A and skin health. Now let's go to Russia for a skin salve: Mix equal parts of zinc-oxide ointment and lanolin until blended. Add an equal amount of garlic powder, a little at a time. (You don't want the mixture to lump or cake.) When smooth, store in covered jar. Use as required. The zinc-oxide ointment and the lanolin are available at drugstores, and the garlic powder at any grocer's.[27]

Oh, your teenager doesn't want to bother with the "mix" and is somewhat skeptical about the raw potato? Well, if someone came up with a magic-bullet cure for acne, the teenagers of America would have a new hero (guru?). Drugs are available, of course, but we all know there is no drug without side effects. The magic-bullet cure must be totally safe and easy, and 100 percent effective. Since the mechanisms causing acne are so complex and varied, and since emotions play a significant role, it is unlikely that such a "cure" will ever happen.

However, there is help for acne. But it's not a magic bullet and it's not easy. The prescription for a peaches-and-cream complexion is loud and clear in the following excerpts:

☆ *Dr. Jonathan Wright,* Harvard-trained medical columnist:

Acne is preventable and is the result of the malnutrition of civilization, and not an inevitable accompaniment of adolescence. Most acne responds to simple dietary measures, such as:
1) Elimination of all refined sugar, refined flours, artificial flavor, color and preservatives.
2) Positive dietary additions: as much fresh raw vegetables and fruits as possible. [We would caution those eating too many fruits. Our daughter's skin erupts every time she has more than one banana in a day.] Sufficient high-quality protein.
3) Supplements, especially including zinc, essential fatty acids [evening primrose oil and/or a quarter of an avocado daily are excellent sources of essential fatty acids], vitamins A, B, and C.[28]

We appreciate Dr. Wright's outline for abolishing acne, but take exception to his comment that his prospectus involves "simple dietary measures." Lifestyles must be recast, and that's not simple. Effective, yes. Easy, no.

☆ *Emory Thurston,* pioneer in food-health research relationships:

Medicines taken internally have little effect, but the dietary is most important. Certain foods definitely aggravate the condition in many patients. Some of the most common culprits are cola drinks, chocolate, fried and rich foods, sweets, ice cream, and milk. Milk is suspect for two reasons: 1) Many people cannot digest milk properly, thus leaving undigested molecules to lodge in various tissues of the body, which may cause some form of allergy; 2) The female hormones in milk are thought to be a possible cause of acne, especially in males. Although important nutrients are destroyed in pasteurization, apparently these are not.

As many vegetables as possible should be eaten raw. If salad dressing is used, it should be limited to vinegar and a small amount of oil with herbs. [See our oil-free salad dressings in the recipe section.] A good vitamin-mineral supplement is very important and may greatly shorten the period of recovery as well as improve general health. The daily intake of at least 500 milligrams of vitamin C and 50,000 units of vitamin A are a must. X-ray treatments are not recommended. They may give some temporary relief but may do great permanent damage to the skin as well as to internal tissue.[29]

A final tip is one we discovered in an obscure report on acne. We know several people who have tried this, and found it worked wonders: For one or two weeks, consume ½ pint of acidophilus liquid culture twice a day (following each of two meals). Acidophilus culture is a fermented milk product, similar to yogurt, and is available in natural-food stores. The complexion will probably worsen for a short period of time before signs of improvement are visible. This is because of the detoxifying action of the acidophilus—the toxins are rapidly being released through the surface of the skin. After the initial period of the intense doses, follow with a maintenance amount of 2 tablespoons after every meal *forevermore*. If nothing else, health will be immeasurably improved. Acidophilus is a superior food product. If everyone consumed two tablespoons of acidophilus culture after each meal, chances are there would be very little acne and an elevation of general health status.

Eczema

In 1919 an observant doctor noticed that a breastfed infant's eczema occurred after his mother had eaten chocolate. The lesions disappeared when chocolate was eliminated from the mother's diet.[30]

Eczema is a general term for any inflammatory condition involving the skin, marked by redness, itching, oozing, crusting, and later by scaling. Actually it is a common allergic reaction in children. Childhood eczema often begins in infancy, the rash appearing on the face, neck, and folds of elbows and knees. It may disappear by itself when the offending food is removed from the diet, or it may become more extensive and in some instances cover the entire surface of the body. Severe eczema can be complicated by skin infections. A child who suffers eczema may develop some other allergic condition later on— most commonly hay fever or asthma.

Eczema is frequently caused by an allergic sensitivity to foods such as milk, fish, or eggs, or even to dusts, pollens, or similar substances that are inhaled.[31]

There are several theories explaining eczema. One is that it may not be a skin disease exclusively, and could be present regardless of food allergy. Another view is that the role of food allergy in eczema is more important than has ever been realized. Whether or not eczema is accompanied by clear evidence of food allergy, there are things going on in the intestines that are not normal. The researchers describe it as "intestinal mucosal defect."[32]

There is a reduced incidence of eczema in children who are breastfed, and whose diet regimen avoids cow's milk, eggs, and fish. The researchers state that the immune system may be especially vulnerable to the introduction of allergic responses in infancy.[33] In addition, milk and dairy products should be eliminated. This program should be followed for about 6 to 8 weeks, and is best done under doctor's advisement.[34]

Dr. Lendon Smith recommends vitamin A in supplemental form. He says: "To say that 5000 units per day of vitamin A is all that anyone should have makes no sense when signs of vitamin A deficiency are obvious. Everyone is different and everyone has his or her own requirements.[35]

Dr. Carl Pfeiffer has identified white spots on the fingernails with zinc deficiency.[36] In some children, the appearance of white spots signals the onset of eczema. This is a good harbinger of symptoms about to blossom.

Dr. Jonathan Wright outlines the following nutritional supplementation plan for eczema:

1) Chelated zinc, 50 milligrams, 3 tablets daily (do *not* continue taking this large quantity of zinc indefinitely; 6 to 8 weeks is maximum; then cut down amounts).

2) 1000 milligrams of vitamin C, twice daily. Vitamin C is essential for healing.
3) One tablespoon cod-liver oil daily.
4) One tablespoon of vegetable oil daily [we recommend a handful of sunflower seeds to avoid rancidity problems].
5) Pancreatic enzymes—2 tablets with each meal.[37]

Hearing

One almost wonders if the title of this entire chapter should be *"Allergies."* Ear infections are so commonplace, and they too are initiated by allergies—usually to cow's milk![38] Another bit of advice to the parents of a child who has chronic ear infections is to make every effort to eliminate sugar. Sugar suppresses the immune system, thereby reducing the body's ability to fight infections. It's a battle, and the soldiers have been devitalized because of their struggle to metabolize the sugar.[39]

Dr. Paul Yanick is an unusual audiologist who started his career as an engineer. He became a unique hearing specialist because he was determined *not* to spend his life living with the problems the doctors told him were incurable: deafness and tinnitus. Dr. Yanick cured himself, and endless others like himself. He has written a special message for parents expressly for this book.

Hearing: A Nutritional Approach

—by Paul Yanick, Jr.
Like all other childhood sicknesses, hearing loss has its roots in the prenatal and early postnatal period of a child's life. Many chemical pesticides, food additives, saccharin and cyclamates, alcohol, nitrates and BHA and BHT, preservatives, sodium derivatives, DES growth hormones from beef, drugs, caffeine (from coffee, tea, cocoa, cola drinks), and tobacco can penetrate the placental barrier and weaken the baby's vital defense systems and organs. During the baby's early years of life, the consumption of refined, overcooked, sugar-

laden, processed, and other denatured foods will deprive the baby of nutrients so important for growth and development of a strong healthy body.

A baby's liver and kidneys in the prenatal state are not sufficiently developed to remove potentially toxic chemicals and substances and to protect against unnecessary chemical invasion. Consequently, if a genetic weakness exists and manifests itself in the hearing mechanism, hearing loss may occur in the post-natal period and throughout life.

Although there is probably some genetic component in all disease processes, the extent of this component varies considerably depending upon the complex interactions that occur between genetics and the environment.

Genetics determine the detailed potentialities of the hearing organ's ability to carry on its intricate and complex functions, *provided the necessary nutrients are supplied.* Although parents of many children with ear problems are told by doctors that their child's hearing loss is hereditary and that nothing can be done to help it or prevent it from getting worse, *it is not impossible to improve these hearing-related problems and prevent ear disease.*

Contrary to the idea which often prevails, ear disease itself is very seldom caused solely on a hereditary basis. Often, the actual causes, i.e., stressor agents, other organ weaknesses, biochemical imbalances, nutrient deficiencies, and metabolic abnormalities, etc., are hereditary. Despite the result of inheritance, environments can be changed or altered to prevent the further progression of hearing loss—and many times these changes will even reverse the process of ear disease.

MIDDLE EAR PROBLEMS

Middle ear malfunctions are the most common cause of hearing loss in infants and children. Often, fluid and/or mucus will accumulate in the middle ear space, causing a hearing loss, earaches, and pressure or fullness in the middle ear. When this condition becomes chronic there is danger of the eardrum rupturing from the expansion of fluid pressure in the middle ear. Generally, these middle ear infections become a recurrent problem for which repeated surgical punctures of the eardrum and long-term ingestions of antibiotics and decongestants are the standard medical treatment. Since the tissues of the middle ear intermittently undergo destruction and scarring during each episode of middle ear infections, it is critical that all precautions are taken in regard to a child's nutritional needs.

The outer ear, eardrum, ear bones, muscles, ligaments, joints, and bony cavities are all delicately molded and must perform in perfect balance to deliver effective sound vibrations to the inner ear. All these parts of the ear demand nutrients for their optimal function. Hearing loss can occur from a multitude of malfunctions with any one part of the ear. Good nutrition, exercise, and diet can prevent many forms of outer and middle ear conditions that nowadays require surgical operations and medications.

Mucus present in the middle ear space is often a reaction of toxicity. Mucus is used by the body as a method of entrapping a potentially harmful substance to prevent it from penetrating deeper into the body and as a medium for expelling this substance from the body. Often, the body responds to ingestion of a particular food with the production of mucus because that food contains some substance the body recognizes as potentially harmful or toxic. For this reason, allergies are often considered by physicians as being involved in middle ear infections. However, it is my experience that the so-called allergic response is often the result of an overload of undigested proteins and foods and/or toxins in the system.

The lymphatic system plays a major role in the removal of toxins from the body, and fights infection. The white blood cells, called lymphocytes, circulate in and out of the lymphatic system, and they help destroy foreign particles like bacteria, viruses, and parasites. In addition, mucus accumulations in the body must be carried off by the lymph fluids. The colon is the principal site of lymphatic toxin and mucus elimination and in many cases long-term recurrent middle ear infections in children are due to constipation and/or excess mucus accumulated in the colon. Mucus in the colon is a result of an overloaded lymphatic system due to poor diet and ingestion of too many mucoid-forming foods. Dietary changes by far are the most effective treatment for mucus buildup anywhere in the body.

We are grateful to Dr. Yanick for this dissertation on the correlation between hearing problems and the nutrition of your child.

Anemia

On an adequate diet, only about 10 to 20 percent of the iron content is absorbed. This is not always enough to meet requirements, so other sources of iron are needed. In nature's wisdom, iron is stored by the body (mainly in the bone marrow). However, the amount is not always sufficient to meet the demand. The relatively small amounts of iron in the diet and low stores of iron are often not enough for the greatly increased requirements of iron for *growth*.[40]

It is virtually impossible for an inadequate diet to be lacking in one nutrient alone. In most instances the quality of the diet is poor because of a lack of a particular food or food group which may be the only source of *several* essential nutrients. For example, green leaves provide the precursor of vitamin A, vitamin C, and riboflavin; cereals are sources of vitamins from the B group.[41]

Nutritional anemia may occur as a result of deficiency in iron, vitamin B_{12} or folates (part of the B-complex). Iron deficiency is the commonest variety of nutritional anemia in children, especially between the ages of 6 months and 3 years. And once again, we indict cow's milk: Milk is a poor source of iron. Human milk contains more iron than cow's milk, but more importantly, the iron in human milk is more easily absorbed by the baby.

The effects of iron-deficiency anemia may be varied. The anemic child is fatigued for long periods of time. Attention spans are reduced, as are alertness and learning capacity. Phytate in cereals and phosphates in milk diminish iron absorption.

Iron needs are increased during puberty for boys and girls due to the sudden growth spurts and excessive bleeding at menstruation in girls. It is essential to feed iron-rich foods during this time. Foods that contain iron are beans, legumes, peas and green leafy vegetables, raw fish, whole fresh eggs, cereals, potatoes and other root vegetables. Natural sources of folic acid (deficiencies of which, as stated, can also cause anemia) are dark green leafy vegetables, dried dates, cauliflower, asparagus, liver, kidney, and brewer's yeast.[42]

The most vulnerable time for anemia? Those periods of life when the requirements for nutrients are increased because of the demands of growth.[43]

Celiac

"There is a kind of chronic indigestion which is met with in persons of all ages, yet is especially apt to affect children between one and five years old. . . . Signs of the disease are yielded by the feces . . . the food having undergone putrefaction rather than concoction. . . . Error in diet may perhaps be a cause." This treatise on "Celiac Affection" was published in 1888.[44] It took half a century or more to recognize that gluten in wheat causes these problems, which include flatulence, weight loss, weakness, and diarrhea. Once wheat is eliminated from the diet, all symptoms disappear.[45] However, treatment with a gluten-free diet must be a lifelong practice. Other grains possessing injurious gluten properties are barley, rye and oats. Because of the fact that so many foods contain wheat (see listings in allergy section), most sensitive children fail to keep a strict, gluten-free diet.[46] If your child is doing well on such a diet, it is not in your child's best interest to reintroduce the gluten.[47]

After a long duration of celiac disease, vitamin B_{12} absorption decreases.[48] Therefore, it is especially significant to be sure that B_{12} foods are part of the celiac child's diet.

Isn't it nice to know there is a disease state that can be relieved without drugs? When gluten is avoided, there is complete remission of the clinical disease, and the abnormalities causing the difficulties are reversed.[49] (Celiac disease is also called nontropical sprue.)

Want some very good news? The incidence of celiac disease in childhood is falling. This is directly related to changes in infant feeding practices occurring in the mid-1970's. The increased prevalence of breastfeeding, thereby reducing the challenge from cow's milk protein too early, and the later introduction of gluten into the diet, may all be important factors in this observed change.[50]

Folic acid deficiency is very common in children with celiac disease. Intestinal malabsorption seems to be the main cause of folic acid deficiency in celiac children over one year of age.[51] Foods containing folic acid are: liver, dark-green, leafy vegetables, asparagus, lima beans, kidney, nuts, whole-grain cereals, and lentils.[52]

Chicken Pox

Chicken pox is nutrient-depleting. Dr. Cathcart, of the University of California in San Francisco, treats his chicken pox patients with massive doses of vitamin C. It's important to remember that pollutants, aspirin, and several other medications cause a loss of vitamin C.[53] It is especially necessary not to smoke in the presence of your children when they are afflicted with such a disorder. We have already discussed the fact that cigarette smoke is an ascorbic acid thief.

Large doses of vitamin C should always be accompanied by calcium, which seems to reduce unpleasant effects. In fact, one of the easiest ways of administering ascorbic acid is to use calcium ascorbate in powdered form, which can easily be mixed in juice or water.

If your child has an appetite, every morsel of food should be of optimum quality. Include concentrated vegetable juice (freshly expressed), dark greens, millet, etc.

Chicken pox is a virus, usually lasting about a week. Slight fever and superficial eruptions are characteristic of chicken pox. If itching is severe, sponging, or bathing with herbal mixtures such as golden seal or burdock root is very helpful. The expression of the skin eruptions are actually toxins that the body is giving off. In addition, avoid constipating foods.

A bath, as warm as the child can comfortably tolerate, will help the child perspire and encourages a faster skin breakout. This will shorten the sick period by a number of days. The folk remedy that our grandmother taught us still works best: After the bath, wrap the child in warm nightclothes *while still wet*, and tuck him or her into bed. Your child will stay warm for many hours. This actually generates an artificial fever, which facilitates the healing process.[54]

Colds and Flu

If a child has *repeated* infections, the reasons may be:

1) Allergy.
2) Low nutrient levels.

3) Immune difficulties.[55]

Seek professional help from persons schooled in getting at *causes.* But right now your child is sick. Here are general rules for handling bouts of respiratory and flu attacks:

1) Get rid of constipation.
2) Ply with nutrients.
3) Relieve symptoms with natural methods.

Let's explore these beneficial tactics.

1) Constipation

Constipation is discussed later in this chapter.

2) Ply with Nutrients

If Linus Pauling and Irwin Stone have their way with vitamin C, the cliché "A cold lasts a week if you treat it, and seven days if you don't" will be outdated. Yes, a cold usually lasts about seven days, but consider these reports on colds and viral infections:

☆ Just as vitamin C will hasten recovery of chicken pox, so will it be beneficial in fighting any infection. Many studies show that at the very least it will *shorten the course* of common virus infections.[56]
☆ Large doses of vitamin C act as *antihistamines* and help reduce cold and allergy symptoms.[57]
☆ Vitamin C is said to *inactivate* some viruses.[58]
☆ Laboratory animals and humans may produce more *infection-fighting white cells* there are adequate levels of vitamin C to help things along.[59]

Dr. Robert Atkins recommends the combination of vitamin C with vitamin A. He suggests large doses of vitamin C every hour and a half, and large doses of vitamin A—all to be continued for five days. He cuts the dosage down to one-half after the initial five days, continuing *another* five days on the reduced dose.[60]

o   o   o

We hesitate to suggest specific quantities because so much depends on 1) how much vitamin C and vitamin A the child has been getting, and 2) how severe the illness is. Experience and judgment are helpful here. Just remember that for a short period of time, there is no harm done, and most probably incredible benefit. The recommended daily allowance of 60 milligrams of vitamin C is sufficient to prevent scurvy, but it is not enough for optimal health, or for the prevention and speedy recovery of colds.[61]

Individual thresholds of vitamin C are usually reached when stools become loose. Should this occur, lower the dose. But flatulence may also present itself for another reason: It could be precipitated by the *acid* part of ascorbic acid tablets. Once again, calcium ascorbate powder minimizes stomach upsets. Another word of caution: Reduce large doses of C *gradually,* even after your patient is in tiptop shape.

As for vitamin A, symptoms of overdose are usually reversible simply by discontinuing the vitamin. The chances of overdose when taking vitamin A for a short period of time are unlikely.

In addition to the vitamin C and vitamin A information, the following nutrient reports are worth noting:

☆ Zinc-deficient children are prone to infections, including viruses.[62]
☆ The body's need for folic acid is increased during times of stress and disease.[63]

Animals refrain from eating during sieges of illness. Your child probably won't have an appetite, either, but it's not difficult to encourage sips of water in which vitamin C powder has been dissolved. You can also simmer vegetables (all kinds, but be sure to include dark, leafy greens), and feed the liquid vegetable broth to your child. This is a powerful nutrient potion. When health is somewhat regained, offer lots of water (not juices, but *water*), increase servings of dark-green, leafy vegetables, and reduce intake of meat and dairy products.[64]

Sprouted seeds and grains are excellent sources of vitamin C. Green peppers have more vitamin C than oranges, and they are an especially good source of vitamin C in winter months.[65]

o   o   o

According to studies at the University of London, caffeine is able to raise body temperature or block the fever-reducing properties of aspirin. Caution! Caffeine is found in regular tea (check the herb tea labels—a few do have caffeine), and colas. So the old-fashioned fever antidote of tea-and-aspirin is a washout!

A marvelous remedy for congestion, which will require supervision, is the facial steambath. Heat a quart or two of water in a large pot. After the water boils, throw lots of herbs into it. Anything you have on hand will do. Lower heat, and let simmer, covered, for 10 to 15 minutes. Remove pot to table. Make a towel tent over your child's head and the pot, being sure that your child is at least 8 inches from the steam that will emanate from the pot. Or, instead of a towel, you can use a small umbrella. Tell your child to breathe deeply. The herbal inhalant will help soothe the respiratory tract and ease the dry, hacking feeling in the throat. When steam quiets down, shake the pot a bit, and it will start up again. A ten-minute steaming will relieve congestion and is also an incredible calmant.

Dian Dincin Buchman, noted herbal researcher, recommends the following procedure for infants with colds: Bruise 2 ounces of anise seeds in a mortar; place them in a pitcher, and pour 2 cups of boiling water over the seeds. Steep this for 15 minutes, cool and strain. Feed the liquid to the infant in teaspoon doses. Use 1 teaspoon for a one-year-old; up to 3 teaspoons for children over 4 years of age.[66]

    Dr. Buchman's relief for a sore throat: apply an apple cider vinegar compress to the throat, and bind it with a larger wool compress.[67]

Herb teas are helpful. Children do not always like them, but among the favorites are the peppermint and orange and lemon mixtures. Buy a package of cinnamon sticks, and place one in each cup of tea. This imparts a pleasant cinnamon flavor and an appealing touch. Cinnamon covers up unpleasant odors, and for this reason it is used frequently in herbal medicine. It also happens to be helpful in diarrhea, and folklore says it helps children who are bedwetters or have difficulty sleeping. It's also an antinausea aid. So in addition to adding a festive touch to the tea, there are many advantages.[68]

    If you cannot get cinnamon sticks, sprinkle ground cinnamon into the tea. Be sure there are no additives (sugar) in the brand you have on hand.

Cinnamon, by the way, is also available in oil form. At the turn of the century, English physicians prescribed five drops of true cinnamon oil to a tablespoon of water. Dose: several times daily at the very onset of the flu epidemic. This remedy is effective preceding the onset of the illness.[69]

(If your herb boxes have been sitting on your shelf more than six months, discard them, and buy fresh containers. And don't store them near your stove.)

IN CONCLUSION

Many nutrition researchers believe that colds and flu only strike those people whose resistance has been dissipated. If you see smoke coming out of a window, you can close the window, but that won't stop the fire. Obviously, you can also put the fire out. That's the difference between saying, "Oh, well, these things happen to children, so we'll let the illness run its course," *or* saying, "Let's confront the cause."

Dental Decay

What illness afflicts about 98 percent of the population to some degree? Dental decay! How many cavities does an average 17-year-old have? 8.7! (And 20 percent have cavities in one-half or more of their teeth!)[70, 71]

Our children never used toothpaste. We taught them to wet their toothbrushes with warm water, and brush properly. They followed the brushing with a thorough taping or flossing between each tooth. A gentle water spray completes the tooth-care regimen.

A house guest asked our daughter Kathi for toothpaste. (She was about three years old at the time.) Kathi's response was, "Why do you want tooth paste? Are your teeth loose?"

It should be noted that we defied heredity. We both have endless fillings in our mouths. The grandparents have no cavities because they have no teeth. However, the children are *cavity-free* (without benefit

of fluorides). This is just one example of how heredity may be inter-
cepted. Tendencies may be inherited; yet we are discovering that because nature tends to the normal, weak traits do not have to surface—
if you supply the tools of the trade: a cornucopia of nutrients.

Dr. Jerome Mittelman, who practices preventive dentistry in New
York City, has prepared this statement for us:

The Truth About Sugar and
Dental Disease

—by Dr. Jerome Mittelman

A number of studies have established that the most important thing
we can do for children to prevent or stop dental disease is to keep
them away from sugar.

Unfortunately many people, including health professionals, don't
seem to want to confront this fact. A great deal of money is being
spent for dental research aimed at finding ways to stop dental disease
without giving up sugar. Researchers are working on vaccines against
the bacteria that are involved in the decay process—a dangerous and
misguided approach if there ever was one! Others are trying to rank
sugar-containing foods according to how cavity-producing they are in
comparison to one another—to see what we can get away with eating.
This research is being sponsored by, among others, manufacturers of
candy and presweetened cereals.

The advice that parents usually get is that if children cut down
on sweets, particularly sticky ones, and brush right after eating them,
they'll be all right. Let's look at what happens, or *doesn't* happen
when you brush after eating. The sugar is taken up right away by
germs in plaque that forms under the gums and between the teeth,
where the brush can't reach. As the late Dr. Robert Barkley said, "You
could brush between bites and it still wouldn't stop decay." Also, as
you eat sugar, it's absorbed from the stomach and goes into the bloodstream, producing far-reaching effects on the body. One of these effects is to change the circulation *within* the tooth so that it becomes
prone to decay. So brushing after eating something sweet isn't going
to have very much effect. As for cutting down on sweets, the average

American child eats so much sugar that merely cutting down, even to one-fourth the usual intake, leaves six or more teaspoons a day in the diet—too much!

The average American family would be shocked to see an actual analysis of how much sugar their children consume each day. Most of it is hidden in foods they eat, not added at the table, in which case they would be aware of how much the children were using. Here are some estimates of hidden sugar in foods:

Cookies, candy—1 to 3 teaspoons per cookie or piece of candy
Puddings, gelatin desserts—4 teaspoons
Ice cream, flavored yogurt, chocolate milk—6 teaspoons
Regular sodas, 12-oz. can—9 teaspoons
Pie (one regular slice)—10 to 14 teaspoons
Pie with ice cream, frosted cake—18 to 20 teaspoons
Ice cream sundae, or cake with ice cream and sundae topping—24 teaspoons

Some health-conscious parents have switched to honey, fructose, raw sugar, molasses, or maple syrup in the hope that these would be more healthful than regular sugar. They are, with the exception of raw sugar, but still can be used to a certain extent by decay-producing bacteria, and a load of concentrated carbohydrate is still going to affect the metabolism of the tooth. The answer is to use these somewhat healthier sweeteners only occasionally and in small quantities, especially if a child has active dental disease and is getting cavities.

Regular and thorough brushing and flossing, regular check-ups, a healthy diet with sufficient protein, whole grains, fresh fruits and vegetables, vitamin and mineral supplements, are all important for dental health—but without a strict limitation on sugar and other concentrated sweeteners, kids aren't going to have healthy teeth.

—JSM

CAUTIONS

☆ Oral irrigating devices do not eliminate plaque.
☆ Although a mouthwash will temporarily freshen breath, it does not remove plaque and cannot prevent decay or gum disease.
☆ Bad breath is usually a sign of poor health.

☆ *The Journal of Prosthetic Dentistry* discusses the effect of topical application of fluoride on composite resin restorations. If your child has had a tooth filled in the last few years, he or she probably has a resin restoration. This is the popular white filling that has replaced mercury fillings now considered dangerous. When fluoride is applied on the surface of resin-filled teeth, it may actually dissolve the fillers. Pitted or roughened surfaces are created, which could then become stained, and lead to increased plaque accumulation. This could, in turn, excite gingivitis. Brushing the teeth with fluoride-containing dentifrices is one way to bring on this undesired domino effect.

☆ *The American Journal of Obstetrics and Gynecology* cites a study involved with the placental transfer of fluoride in pregnancy. According to the researchers, high levels of fluoride can result in high-output renal failure. Their study reveals rapid transfer of the fluoridation across the placenta, with the baby winding up with more of the fluoride than the mother in a matter of *one minute.*

☆ Inform your physician or dentist as soon as possible if you notice white, brown, or black spots on your children's teeth. This may be a sign of too much fluoride.

☆ *The United States Pharmacopeia,* an official publication used by registered pharmacists and recognized by the FDA, reports these possible side effects from fluoride: diarrhea, drowsiness, nausea, stomach cramps or pain, watery eyes, constipation, skin rash, weight loss— among other symptoms.

Just as no person is an island, sugar alone is not responsible for cavities—although it does play a leading role. Additional factors may be immunological and certainly other dietary components.

Constipation

Jonathan Swift, the author of *Gulliver's Travels,* wrote a little book in 1733 in which he described different types of stools. Then as now the subject was so taboo that he did not sign his full name to the published material. But then as now, his description of stools representing health and those representing ill health were most appropriate. He describes the "bad" guys as being similar to balls, buttons, or bullets.[72]

Constipation is a signal that your child's diet is not optimal. Here are many suggestions that will not only relieve constipation, but will enhance the diet:

☆ Timing and constipation may be related. Try serving a whole-grain breakfast (including cereal, whole-grain bread and liquids) at least one-half hour before your child leaves for school. This may mean getting up earlier, but isn't it worth it if you can ensure health for the rest of your child's life? It usually takes about 30 minutes after such a meal for the elimination process to start. Once the child is on his or her way to school, it may not be convenient to visit the bathroom. This is a very important aspect of constipation. Delay often results in a more compacted stool, and sets a pattern of ignoring the "urge"— leading to chronic constipation.[73]

☆ All refined products should be replaced with whole-grain products.

☆ Grated carrot in a salad is an excellent anti-constipation measure. So is chewing on lots of raw fibrous vegetables.

☆ Cow's milk is one of the most common constipating agents for children. Try eliminating milk and see what happens.

☆ The same acidophilus that is so helpful for acne works wonders for proper bowel function.

☆ Fruits that are most effective are raw apples, pears, fresh pineapples, and fresh figs. The seeds of figs act as an intestinal broom, sweeping waste materials through with a laxative effect. Buy *fresh* figs, not the dried or syrupy variety.

☆ Use foods with polyunsaturated oils, which are avocados, sunflower seeds, sesame seeds (use Protein-Aide sesame seeds—they are mechanically hulled); and flaxseeds. Sprinkle the seeds generously on other foods (salads, cereals, etc.). Psyllium seeds, available in natural-food stores, are especially beneficial.

☆ Raw spinach added to salads has a slightly laxative action.

☆ Lack of liquids is a contributing factor. Encourage water consumption. Introduce buttermilk and herb teas at an early age. The teas that are especially helpful are: fern, caraway seed tea, chamomille, and golden seal.

☆ Constipation may have an emotional basis. Teaching relaxation methods early in life is another gift you can bestow on your children.[74]

☆ Unprocessed bran has the highest fiber content of any food product. However, it is not a whole, natural food, and there are some cautions. If you decide to use bran, soak the bran overnight, or at least for a few hours. Excessive bran can cause its own set of nutritional and digestive problems, such as failure to absorb all of the essential nutrients in food. It is preferable to eat bran in the form of whole-grain products and to increase roughage by consuming fruits and vegetables that are not peeled or processed.

Hippocrates, in 430 B.C., said, "You people, complaining of your health, should pass large, bulky motions after every meal, and that to insure this you should eat abundantly of whole meal bread, vegetables and fruits . . ."[75] So what else is new?

Diarrhea

Of course we want to stop the diarrhea as quickly as possible, but we also want to get to the cause. Diarrhea could be a symptom of many diseases.

Diarrhea is defined as the passage of unformed stools with marked or excessive frequency. It's often seen when the child cannot tolerate milk sugar and other sugars. Diarrhea may also be caused by the presence of poisonous byproducts of bacteria or unabsorbed fats, or in response to celiac disease, wheat-gluten sensitivity, stress or emotional problems. Sometimes diarrhea can be the result of other food allergies. As soon as the offending food has been digested or eliminated, the diarrhea disappears. Eating unripe fruits and indigestible substances can bring on the affliction. Perhaps because it is a symptom of so many disease states, diarrhea ranks second only to respiratory diseases as the cause of nonsurgical pediatric admissions to hospitals.[76]

In the infant, diarrhea may be caused by formula that is too concentrated or rich in carbohydrates, or by overfeeding. Check with your pediatrician.

Beware of drugs for toddler diarrhea. One in particular has caused drowsiness, irritability, unacceptable behavior and personality changes. If your doctor is prescribing a drug for diarrhea, why not ask him if there is another method of control?[77]

According to Dr. Fima Lifshitz, Professor of Pediatrics at Cornell

University Medical College, and Marjorie Marks-Katz, nutritionist in pediatric endocrinology, traditional measures for checking diarrhea (such as fasting, and gradual resumption of diet with fluids and soft, bland foods) are not valid. Their explanation of why these modalities are *myths* has been prepared for this chapter:

> Bowel rest has long been a traditional treatment in diarrheal disease. Fasts, or clear liquid diets of up to 72 hours "to provide rest" for the gastrointestinal tract have been used by doctors as well as by the lay public. However, at present, there is decreasing emphasis on such food restriction. In addition to generalized undesirable metabolic effects, lack of or inadequate oral intake may cause alterations in intestinal absorption and intestinal enzyme activities. When a child's nutritional status has been jeopardized by poor intake or excessive nutrient losses due to diarrhea, nutritional therapy becomes even more important for the patient's recovery.
>
> The "BRATT" diet for the treatment of diarrhea in children was not so named because of someone's perverse sense of humor. "BRATT" stands for "bread, rice, applesauce, toast and tea." The diet consists of repetitive feedings of applesauce, bananas, whole-wheat toast with jelly, rice, and tea with sugar. Though this has been a popular mode of nutritional therapy for many years, there is no scientific rationale for using this regime. True, the diet contains apples and bananas which are rich in pectin, a substance which may have "anti-diarrheal" properties. However, this diet is too high in carbohydrate, containing 318 grams. And it's too low in protein and fat, containing *only* 15 grams, and 3.5 grams respectively. It provides 75 to 150 milligrams of caffeine per cup of tea. Therefore, the high osmolality of such a high carbohydrate diet, plus the large caffeine load, can actually result in diarrhea.
>
> The preferred nutritional treatment of diarrhea should be a diet as close to the normal as possible. The maintenance of fluid and electrolyte balance in the child is vital. In most instances this can be attained by increasing oral fluid intake as soon as diarrhea begins. Fasting should only be used as a mode of therapy when complications prevent the child from maintaining oral intake. Oral feedings should be resumed as soon as they are tolerated to help maintain bowel function. Furthermore, it has been shown that children who are *fed* recover sooner and with a better body weight than those who are fasted.[78]

It takes time for new medical knowledge to catch up. Traditional practices linger. You will find the BRATT regimen printed in medical books published *this* year. However, score one for *Grandma*. Her measures, practiced for centuries, have been shown to be effective. Among them is the use of *herbal* teas. The following are helpful for diarrhea: red raspberry, yarrow, oak bark, bayberry bark, garden sage, nettle, strawberry leaves, ginger, and plantain (not the banana, but the herb).[79] Binding foods are: brown rice and baked potatoes. Try apple peel (grandma's remedy—it works.)[80]

Headache

Causes of headache could be: infections, pollution, food additives, exposure to fluorescent light, stress, poor eyesight, toothaches, sinus infections, hunger, backaches, lack of sleep, allergies, consumption of MSG, parents' cigarette smoke, illness (mild; fever), or even sudden increase in salt.[81] A combination of stress factors may make a headache worse. For example, consuming a glass of milk and an orange as an evening snack, and then facing a sports competition the next day will intensify symptoms—if these are stress factors in your child's life.

Try relaxation modalities, such as sitting under a blue light, or taking footbaths. (Immerse both feet in a tub or a basin of cold water for 15 minutes as often as needed.)[82]

If you have made changes in eating lifestyle, and your child still gets recurrent headaches, chances are they are allergic reactions. On a good diet, a child is better able to cope with stress. Record everything your child is eating, and take note of headache experiences. You will see correlations. This is so much more accurate than any of the skin, sublingual or other kinds of allergy tests. Again—you have to be your own doctor. Needless to say, if *severe* symptoms persist, see your physician, and report your findings. Your observations coupled with the doctor's expertise should solve the problem.

If the diary fails to work, you might try eliminating foods reported to be the most frequent cause of allergy headaches. They are (in descending order of frequency): wheat, eggs, tea, coffee, milk, chocolate, beef, corn, sugar, yeast, citrus fruit and cheese. If Mom, Dad, or a grandparent happens to have high blood pressure, that relative should join the child in the elimination diet. The bonus? The blood pressure may just normalize![83, 84]

Digestive Disorders

Other than overprocessed rich nonfoods, the food items most often associated with gas production are onions, cooked cabbage, raw apples, radishes, and beans (especially pinto and soy beans). Flatulence caused by beans can be reduced by sprouting beans before cooking. This, however, requires advance planning.

An effective infant digestive aid may be prepared by soaking 1 to 2 teaspoons of caraway seeds in 1 cup of cold water for 6 hours. The seeds should be bruised first. After the soaking period, strain the water, and give the infant the strained water up to 3 times a day, 1 teaspoon at a time.[85]

Menstruation

Dysmenorrhea is menstrual discomfort. It is usually due to uterine muscle activity, but the cause of this activity is not entirely understood. Severe cramps indicate excessive contraction. Muscles hurt when they don't have adequate oxygen supplies. So, a tight cervical canal might be aggravated by excessive muscle contraction, and might retard the outflow of a hormone present in mucus secretions of the uterine lining. Heavy periods can be due to a shift in these hormone levels. The hormones are called *prostaglandins,* and they help control the contractability of muscle tissue. Many teenagers have pain because they have a higher level of "bad guy" prostaglandins, and not enough of the helpful "good guy" prostaglandins. Prostaglandins may also contribute to blood circulation to the uterus organ itself. If menstrual problems are caused by prostaglandin malfunctions, a good supplement called evening primrose oil often alleviates the discomfort by supplying essential fatty acids in a form which is easy to assimilate. This in turn promotes the right prostaglandin balance.[86]

Premenstrual tension occurs when the body stores greater amounts of salt and water just before the menstrual flow starts. A temporary imbalance between estrogen and progesterone takes place. Breast tenderness can be caused by fluid retention and altered hormone levels.

Sometimes irregular periods are promoted because of sudden weight loss (crash diets) or extreme emotional stress. Undernutrition delays the onset of menstruation and interferes with regulation. Obesity can cause irregular cycles and increased blood loss. Jogging can lead to a reduction in circulating hormones with consequent cessation of menstruation.[87]

There are normal iron losses during menstruation that are constant for each female, but varies from one to another. Inadequate iron levels are due to inadequate iron intake—not to menstruation. Iron foods are: lean meat, dark leafy greens, whole grains, liver and other organ meats, legumes, and shellfish. B vitamins and protein are needed by the liver to convert hormones necessary for the menstrual process. Bioflavonoids have been shown to be helpful. In some cases, premenstrual depression subsides with vitamin B_6. Ascorbic acid is lowest during menstruation. Therefore additional vitamin C may be in order. One study shows that girls taking zinc along with vitamin B_6 have normal cycles within 3 months.

Reducing sodium intake is helpful. Encourage your teenager to eliminate salt, soy sauce and processed foods, and to eat potassium-rich foods (bananas, etc.), in addition to drinking lots of water, and supplementing with B-complex, such as brewer's yeast. Calcium and magnesium supplements have also been suggested as helpful. Further recommendations: a very high bulk diet which includes whole grains and raw vegetables. (Law of Choice #1 does it again!)

To alleviate pain, try back massage, hot pads, tub soaks, and rest.

Conclusion

Hippocrates' *Physician's Oath* states that "Healing is a matter of time, but it is sometimes also a matter of opportunity." Time takes care of itself. We hope *you* will provide your children with the best healing opportunities.

Chapter 7

THE KITCHEN IN TRANSITION

Then all of us prepare to rise
And hold our bibs before our eyes.
And be prepared for some surprise
When father carves the duck.
        —Ernest Vincent Wright,
        When Father Carves the Duck,
                Stanza 1

Are you a beginner? Are you on your way? Are you a purist? Here are recipes for you—wherever you are on the good food continuum. Our best advice for the tenderfoot is to make changes slowly. If you are already on your way, but not yet at the top, there's room for improvement. If you're a purist, you're a winner, and you'll be delighted with new ideas to add to your existing collection.

We learn from vestiges of very early civilizations that food was an intrinsic part of culture: The importance of a favorable experience with food was considered equal to enjoyment derived from any other intellectual or esthetic happening. Therefore, the serving of food was an *art form.* Color, shape, harmony, texture, combination, even aroma were all vitally significant. If the term "holistic" had been popular in the long ago, it would have been stated that it was culturally inherent for food to fit the holistic picture. The appearance of food was not divorced from its nutrition—the *art* of dispensing a meal was as important as the *biochemistry* of its nourishment.

How can *we* apply this concept? Consider the effect of green peas right out of the can (the vision is one of dullness, mushiness, and wishy-washyness) with the esthetics of green peas right out of the shell (the imagery perceived now includes bright color, crispness, and pungency). Reflect on the odor permeating a household in which bread is baking compared with the non-sensing (no pun intended) experience of ripping off the plastic wrapper of a store-bought loaf. As Archie Bunker would say, "Case closed." However, the implementation of new ideas in the kitchen is time-consuming, and most of us are double-parked much of the day. Once again: *That which is familiar becomes convenient.* Well, *the unfamiliar can become the order of the day.* But *the transition should occur bit by bit by bit* (barring emergency needs).

Kitchen Mission: Nutrition

In your kitchen mission for nutrition, these general hints are helpful:

1) Purchases and preparations should follow Laws of Choice #1 and #2, wherever possible. This means your children will be eating foods that are more "natural" and which contain fewer contaminants. Based on these principles, recipes are almost unnecessary. When we study other cultures, we learn that a primary diet is the optimal diet; that gourmet cooking is *not* in the best health interest of your family. It has been said that life is simple, but that we make it complicated. So have we made cooking a tough task, yet *it can be so easy.* However, plunking down a plate on which you have placed a green pepper, some carrot sticks and a bouquet of broccoli will not win favor. You'll find *yourself* eating green peppers, carrot sticks, and broccoli bouquets, while the rest of the family has disappeared to the nearest fast-food shelter. To dispel the myth that basic- or primary-food meals are not much more exciting than going out into the field and grazing on clover, purchase a supply of fresh and dried condiments (oregano, thyme, rosemary, etc., etc.—the works). That's hint number one!

2) Use raw certified whole milk if available.

3) Purchase low-sodium baking powder in a natural-food store. That's for "In the Beginning" recipes. Ideally, "Top of the Line" meals should not use any baking powder. The same applies for baking soda.

4) Some of these recipes enlist the services of honey as a sweetening agent. Use raw, unfiltered honey, and include less and less with each subsequent preparation. Bananas and pineapple are sweet enough. After a while, the sweet craving will subside. (It really will.)

5) We recommend Protein-Aide sesame seeds. These are chemical-free, and mechanically hulled. The hull of the sesame seed contains oxalic acid in quantities that have proved to be dangerous.[1] Primitive cultures did not eat the sesame seed hulls.[2] Essential fatty acids are an important nutrient. However, we rarely get enough in our diet, with the exception of a rancid variety as found in many processed salad dressings. These oils may actually damage cells. The best sources of essential fatty acids come from *whole* foods such as sesame seeds.[3]

6) Vanilla extract should be pure. Since most extracts contain additives, refer to the list in the Appendix under *Resources* for special places that sell "honest" products.

7) There are several bouillon and seasoning substitutes on the market. Some are excellent; others have additives. Check labels carefully.

8) If you think beans exist solely for arts-and-crafts projects such as making necklaces or pasting on collages, you probably also think that the bean is a low-status food. How unfortunate! It's time we joined the ranks of the ancient Egyptians who dedicated temples to beans, worshipping them as symbols of life itself. Beans are rich in high-quality protein, are low in fat, contain important minerals, and even have fiber. Beans are the basis for cuisine from simple to elegant the world over. Learn bean cookery. You will be rewarded.

By the way, if you decide you want to prepare a bean casserole for dinner, and have not soaked beans overnight, all is not lost provided dinner is at least a few hours away. The short-cut: boil beans in water for 2 minutes. Soak beans in this water for 2 hours. Then cook according to instructions.

9) Since no preservatives will be used in your home-baked bread, cake or cookie recipes, refrigerate the finished goodies if they are not consumed within a day or two, especially in warm climates.

10) Purchase natural unprocessed cheese made from whole, certified raw milk. (It's available at natural-food stores.)

11) Use only unsweetened coconut. Most commercial brands

contain sugar and/or additives. Untainted coconut is available in natural-food stores, or from the suppliers listed in the *Resource* section of the Appendix.

But why not have fun with a fresh coconut? Your children will love the experience. Pierce two of the three eyes with a nail, drain the coconut milk (which everyone will adore), break the coconut open, serve some pieces in chunks, and grate the rest. Store the shreds in a tightly sealed container in the refrigerator.

12) Buy oil in small quantities. Look for oil that has been subjected to the least amount of processing. With the exception of olive oil, keep refrigerated. To counteract oxidation, express the contents of a vitamin E capsule into the bottle of oil. Vitamin E is an *anti-oxidant.*

13) Don't discard old cookbooks. Study the stages of good health progression in our recipes, and apply the same changes to your vintage favorites *as your family's palate becomes more educated and ready to accept the innovations.*

14) You will note that wheat germ is not included in "Top of the Line" recipes. Wheat germ is a fractured food product: It is only *part* of the wheatberry. Although wheat germ enhances a poor diet, there are better ways of getting nutrients on "Top of the Line" programs.

15) Trays or jars of sprouting wheatberries should be a kitchen staple. Sprouted wheatberries are crunchy and sweet, two aspects of taste children adore. Add to soups, salads, sandwich spreads, etc. For the gluten-sensitive, be sure to remove any unsprouted seeds. Sprouting erases or at least mitigates problems for those who do have reactions to gluten in grains.

16) Some brands of tamari (soy sauce) contain less salt than others. Check labels. Write to manufacturers if necessary.

17) Soak all dried fruit for at least a few hours, if not overnight. This will rehydrate the fruit, bringing it closer to its natural form, as nature intended.

18) Pizza is served in more mid-Atlantic restaurants than in all of Italy. Although we cannot make the same statement for Oriental foods such as tofu (soybean curd), tempeh (fermented soybean cakes), and miso (soybean or rice paste used for stock), these products are gaining in popularity. They are available in Oriental food stores, in many vegetable markets, in some supermarkets, and in most natural-food stores. It should be obvious that many foods which have been staples for

healthy cultures throughout centuries are nutritious foods. Scientific analysis has labeled tofu a good source of protein, B vitamins and calcium; tempeh as boasting protein and B vitamins including B_{12}, usually available in significant quantities only in animal foods; and miso as rating equally high in these nutrients.[4]

19) The best recipes may not appear in this section because they are so basic. For example, a dinner of lightly steamed vegetables (steam only until the vegetables reach prime color and are still crispy), and steamed fish or chicken, plus a large tossed salad containing 10 or 12 raw ingredients (including sprouts), embellished with whole fruit and nuts for dessert, is one of the ultimates in "Top of the Line" meals. There was a time when friends asked, "How can you work and have a full course dinner?" "We can't," we answered, "We're having bananas and cereal for supper." And then we learned how easy it is to raise the status of basic foods from rank-and-file to aristocracy.

Thomas Henry Huxley has said, "The great end of life is not knowledge, but action."[5] This section of the book explains how to take your new knowledge and translate it into *action*.

The Recipes

Rise and Shine

Let the *real* breakfast of champions step forward! How about hearty, stick-to-the-ribs recipes that will help your kids be winners?

BIRD'S NEST

In the Beginning

6 slices whole-grain bread; 1 tablespoon butter; 6 eggs.

Remove a 3-inch diameter from the center of each piece of bread. Butter pan. Heat bread on one side. Flip bread over and break an egg carefully into the hole in each piece. Season to taste. Toast center portions for children to snack on while breakfast is cooking. Serves 6. (Our children called this the "Framed Egg.")

On Your Way

Use coarse, whole-grain bread, baked with a minimum of sweetening agents.

Top of the Line

Use sprouted whole-grain bread.
Do not toast centers. Use fertile, organic eggs.

GRANOLA

In the Beginning

4 cups rolled oats; 1 cup wheat germ; 1 teaspoon sea salt; 2 teaspoons cinnamon; 2 teaspoons nutmeg; 1 teaspoon allspice; ¾ cup vegetable oil; 1 cup honey; 1 teaspoon vanilla; 1 teaspoon almond extract; 1 cup chopped almonds.

In large bowl combine oats, wheat germ, salt, cinnamon, nutmeg, and allspice. In separate bowl, combine oil, honey, vanilla, and almond extract. Combine both mixtures. Add nuts. Spread in large greased pan; bake at 350° for 20 minutes, stirring frequently. Cool and break into chunks. MAKES 6 CUPS.

On Your Way

Reduce wheat germ to ½ cup. Reduce salt to ½ teaspoon. Reduce oil to ½ cup. Reduce honey to ½ cup. Add ½ cup sesame seeds.

Top of the Line

#1
Eliminate wheat germ and use ¼ cup whole wheat bread crumbs instead. Reduce oil to ¼ cup, and add ¼ cup melted butter. Reduce honey to 1 tablespoon. Add ½ cup raisins, drained, which have soaked in apple juice for several hours. Add 1 cup sprouted wheatberries after mixture has soaked and cooled. (Again: for the gluten-sensitive, remove unsprouted berries.)
#2
2½ cups rolled oats; 1½ tablespoons shredded coconut; 1½ tablespoons sunflower seeds; 3 tablespoons chopped almonds; ½ cup ses-

ame seeds; 3 tablespoons raisins, drained, which have soaked in water several hours; 1 teaspoon cinnamon.

Spread liquid lecithin (break open a capsule) on baking pan. Combine oats, coconut, sunflower seeds, almonds, sesame seeds. Sprinkle on pan in shallow layer. Bake uncovered at 350° about 20 minutes, stirring occasionally. Remove from oven, add raisins and cinnamon. Cool and store in covered jar. MAKES 6½ CUPS.

#3

Add the following mixture to any of the above granola recipes: 1 cup sprouted wheatberries, 1 cup sprouted oats, 1 cup sprouted rice grains, 1 cup sprouted soybeans. Grind and blend into powder. Optional: add 1 raw or lightly cooked egg to this sprouted, powdered blend.

SPROUTED WHEAT CEREAL

In the Beginning

3 cups sprouted wheatberries; ½ cup chopped dried fruit (raisins, apples, etc.), soaked in unsweetened fruit juice; 2 tablespoons raw honey.

Steam sprouted wheatberries and dried fruit in small amount of water until both are tender. *Serves 8.*

On Your Way

Omit honey. Sweeten cereal with stewed strawberries, or peach, pear, or apple juice.

Top of the Line

Use ½ cup sprouted wheatberries and ½ cup sprouted rye berries. Since different grains offer different nutrients, combinations of grains are ideal. Experiment: try 5-grain mixtures, or 7-grain mixtures. Omit all sweetening agents.

BREAKFAST BAR

In the Beginning

6 eggs; 3 cups granola; 1 cup currants, raisins or dates (chopped); ½ cup almonds, chopped fine; ½ cup sesame seeds; ¼ cup sunflower seeds; 1 teaspoon cinnamon.

Beat eggs. Add remaining ingredients; mix well. Batter will be thick. Let mixture sit 15 minutes while oven preheats to 350°. Pour mixture into well-oiled 9-inch-square pan. Press mixture into pan; smooth top. Bake 25 to 30 minutes or until lightly brown and firm. Remove from oven; cut into 1-by-2-inch bars while hot. Remove from pan by loosening edges gently with spatula. Cool. Store in airtight container. MAKES 3 DOZEN.

On Your Way

Reduce chopped fruit to ½ cup.

Top of the Line

Reduce chopped fruit to ½ cup.
Use "Top of Line" granola #3.

The Bread Basket

If you want to keep your children at home, never mind TV computer games or backyard swimming pools. Just permeate the house with the incomparable aroma of bread baking!

WHOLE-GRAIN BREAD

In the Beginning

1 cup water; ¼ cup honey; 1 teaspoon sea salt; ⅓ cup oil; ¾ cup milk; 1 cup wheat germ; 2 tablespoons yeast; ¼ cup lukewarm water; 3 cups whole wheat flour; 3 cups unbleached white flour.

Combine water, honey, salt and oil in saucepan. Heat; stir until blended. Cool to lukewarm and pour into large bowl. Combine wheat germ and milk. Let soak while honey mixture cools. Dissolve yeast in ¼ cup lukewarm water. Add wheat-germ mixture and yeast to liquids in bowl. Stir in flour, kneading last part. Turn onto floured board and knead well until dough is smooth and elastic. Cover with damp cloth. Let rise in warm place 1 hour or until dough doubles in bulk. Punch down, shape into 2 loaves. Place in oiled bread tins. Let rise, covered, 45 minutes. Bake at 400° for 50 minutes. Cool slightly before slicing.

On Your Way

1 tablespoon honey; 1½ cups warm water; 2 teaspoons yeast; 3 cups whole-wheat flour; 1 teaspoon oil (optional).

Mix honey and water and dissolve yeast. Wait until mixture foams. Mix this into flour and oil. Knead and add more flour as needed. Let rise 30 to 40 minutes. Punch down and put in loaf pans; let rise 20 to 30 minutes more. Place in preheated 350° oven. Bake 20 minutes or until golden-brown. (*Note:* If you find breads made of 100 percent whole grains too heavy, try adding some ground popcorn to dough. This lightens texture.)

Top of the Line

1 cup wheatberries; 2 cups water; 2 tablespoons raisins (optional).

Soak wheatberries 15 hours. Drain next day, wet and drain twice daily for 3 days. Put through blender, processor, or juicerator, and mold into loaf. If using raisins or other ingredients, such as dried fruit, nuts, cinnamon, caraway seeds, poppy or sesame seeds, add at this point. Bake at 350° for about 30 minutes. Note: when molding loaf, use oil plus water as needed to thicken. Additional flavors of added ingredients permeate loaf as it sits around.

The Souper Bowl

A bowl of soup can be a hearty meal or a dieter's delight. Either way, a kettle simmering all day on "warm" provides a course or a snack at the ready any time of the day. (Caution: restaurant soup and canned soups are overdosed with salt.)

LENTIL SOUP

In the Beginning

1 16-ounce package lentils; 2 medium onions, sliced; 2 medium carrots, sliced; 1 cup celery, sliced; 1 tablespoon sea salt; ½ teaspoon pepper; ½ teaspoon thyme leaves; 2 bay leaves; 8 cups water; 4 nitrite-free frankfurters, cut in chunks.

1½ hours before serving, rinse lentils in running cold water. Discard any small rocks. In 5-quart saucepot over medium heat, cook lentils and all other ingredients except frankfurters to boiling. Reduce heat to low. Cover. Simmer 1 hour or until lentils are tender. Discard bay leaves. Add frankfurters. Heat through. MAKES ABOUT 11 CUPS OR 6 SERVINGS.

On Your Way

Eliminate salt. Use only 2 frankfurters.

Top of the Line

Eliminate salt. Use only 2 frankfurters. Sprout lentils for 1 or 2 days before cooking. Save a few sprouted lentils to add to soup uncooked just before serving. (See Sprouting instructions.)

MEAL-IN-A-BOWL SOUP

In the Beginning

2 quarts water; small handful whole-wheat spaghetti or spinach noodles; ½ cup each of diced onion, green pepper, celery, carrot, sweet potato, zucchini, mushrooms, squash; 2 tablespoons tamari; dash pepper; oregano; thyme; 1 garlic clove (or crushed garlic).

Bring water to boil. Add noodles. Reduce heat and cover. Cook on low for ½ hour. Add vegetables, tamari, and seasonings. Barely simmer for 1 to 2 hours, or until ready to serve. (If whole garlic clove used, remove clove.) Aroma permeating house is an appetite stimulant.

On Your Way

Use brown rice instead of noodles.

Top of the Line

Sprout brown rice one day before cooking. Add ½ cup of sprouted garbanzos just before serving.

The Main Event

If you don't want your children to ask why nature didn't place the vitamins in the ice cream instead of the parsley, try your hand at some of these recipes.

ORIENTAL BROWN RICE
In the Beginning

1 tablespoon sesame oil; 1 cup raw brown rice; 2 cups water; 1 cup mushrooms; 3 tablespoons additional sesame oil; 1 cup chopped celery; 1 cup chopped green or red peppers; 3 tablespoons tamari; 1 cup diced water chestnuts; 1 cup green peas; 1 cup chopped scallions; 4 cloves mashed garlic; 2 cups bean sprouts; 2 eggs.

Place 1 tablespoon oil in skillet and heat. Add rice slowly, with heat still on, stirring continuously until each grain is coated with oil. (*Note:* This only takes a few minutes, but this unusual step will prevent grains from sticking together. Another method for avoiding grain-stickiness is to place 2 tablespoons of oil into the pot of water in which the rice will cook.) Pour water into another pot. Bring to boil. Add oil-coated rice slowly and cover. Reduce heat to lowest possible setting; cook 30 minutes. An old Chinese rice-cooking rule is: No peeking! (Lifting cover allows steam to escape, and rice will not cook enough.)

Stir-fry mushrooms; set aside. Add remainder of oil and stir-fry celery and pepper (and any other vegetables such as broccoli or zucchini). Stir-fry only until vegetables reach prime color. Add tamari. Add rice and stir entire mixture. Now add water chestnuts, green peas, scallions, garlic, and sprouts. Lightly scramble 2 eggs and toss into mixture. Optional: add 1 or 2 cups of diced chicken or turkey.

On Your Way

Reduce tamari to 1½ teaspoons.

Top of the line

Reduce tamari to ½ teaspoon. Do not sauté any of the vegetables. Add all vegetables in raw state after the rice is cooked.

DELICIOUS MILLET

In the Beginning

2 cups water; 1 cup whole millet; 1 cup chopped sweet onion; 3 tablespoons sesame oil; 1 chopped green pepper; 4 cloves minced garlic; 1 cup chopped mushrooms; 1 cup green peas and/or diced zucchini; 2 ta-

blespoons soy grits; 1 cup finely chopped carrots; ½ teaspoon salt; 3 ta-
blespoons tamari.

Bring water to boil. Add millet; simmer, covered, on low heat, for about 20 minutes. In separate large skillet, lightly sauté onion. Add remaining ingredients, except tamari. Steam, covered, 5 minutes. Add tamari. Stir millet into vegetables. Heat through a few minutes more. Variation: Add natural grated cheese before baking. Bake in 325° oven for 10 to 15 minutes or until top is lightly brown.

On Your Way

Eliminate salt and oil. Sprinkle millet and vegetables with sesame seeds and paprika.

Top of the Line

2 cups water; 1 cup whole millet; dash pepper; handful of sunflower seeds; 2 cloves minced garlic; sesame seeds.

Boil water. Add millet. Lower heat and cook, covered, 15 to 20 minutes or until all water is absorbed. Add dash of pepper, handful of sunflower seeds and garlic. Sprinkle with sesame seeds. Season with only as much tamari as necessary to reach acceptable palatability. Add raw diced vegetables.

MIXED BEAN CASSEROLE

In the Beginning

2 cups red beans; 2 cups kidney beans; 2 cups garbanzo beans (or any combination of these beans); 1 pound ground beef; 1 large onion, chopped; 2 teaspoons dry mustard; ¼ cup water; 3 tablespoons apple cider vinegar; 1 cup tomato sauce; pepper to taste.

Drain beans and save liquid (in case mixture becomes too dry). Place beans in 2½-quart casserole. Mix lightly; set aside. In large skillet, cook ground beef, onions, and garlic until meat is lightly browned. Stir in remaining ingredients. Add skillet mixture to beans in casserole; mix together. Cover; bake about 1 hour in preheated oven, 325°. *Serves 8.*

On Your Way

Eliminate ground beef.

Top of the Line

Eliminate ground beef. Soak beans 24 hours; drain and sprout additional 24 hours.

STUFFED PEPPERS

In the Beginning

4 bell peppers; ¼ pound sliced mushrooms; ¼ cup chopped celery; 2 tablespoons oil; 2 cups cooked brown rice; ½ cup cooked meat, ground, or finely diced chicken; 1 cup vegetable stock; ½ teaspoon basil; ¼ teaspoon pepper.

Cut tops off peppers; remove seeds and pulp. Rinse and drain. Sauté mushrooms and celery in oil until tender. Remove from heat. Add brown rice and meat; stir in stock and seasonings; fill peppers with mixture. Place in deep casserole. Bake 30 minutes at 375°, covered.

On Your Way

Top with grated raw natural cheese made from whole milk. Return to oven briefly. Serve on bed of dark, leafy greens.

Top of the Line

Replace ½ cup of cooked meat with ½ cup of sprouted beans, mashed. (Rice and beans complement each other, creating complete protein when served together.)

VEGETABLE MEDLEY

If your children are not vegetable eaters and have not tasted them in years, one way to get them to be adventurous is to tell them that there is now a new variety that has been grown for better flavor. You are not being entirely dishonest: The vegetables, of course, are the same, but what *is* new is your ability to serve them in tastier fashion. Chances are your children will respond and hopefully will discover that vegetables are not so bad after all!

In the beginning

2 tablespoons oil; 1 minced onion; 1 minced garlic clove; 1 diced celery stalk; 1 chopped apple; 1 cup water; ½ teaspoon sea salt; 1 teaspoon dillweed; 2 cups chopped vegetables, including carrots, squash, and cabbage.

Sauté in oil: onion, garlic, celery, and apple. Add water, salt, dillweed, and vegetables. Stir and cook just crisply done. Serve with brown rice and chopped nuts.

On Your Way

Eliminate salt.

Top of the Line

Eliminate salt. Add 1 cake of cubed tofu to vegetables when sautéing.

TOFU SLOPPY JOES

In the Beginning

1 tablespoon oil; ½ onion, finely minced; a few mushrooms; ½ block of tofu (8 ounces); 1½ teaspoons parsley (save some for decoration); ½ teaspoon each of oregano and sweet basil; ½ clove minced garlic; 8 ounces spaghetti sauce; 4 muffins; ¼ pound grated mozzarella cheese.

Heat pan with oil; sauté onions and mushrooms, until translucent, but not brown. Push aside. Add more oil. Crumble tofu into oiled section of pan. Mix with vegetables. Add spices: parsley, basil, oregano, garlic. Mix. Keep stirring. This is a fast procedure. Stir until steaming stops. Curds will get bigger and firmer. Add spaghetti sauce. Stir. Toast muffins. Pour mixture on muffins and place under broiler after sprinkling cheese. (Parmesan or Romano may also be used) on top. Omit cheese for lactose-intolerant children.

On Your Way

Use homemade or sugar-free and preservative-free spaghetti sauce.

Top of the Line

Use homemade or sugar-free and preservative-free spaghetti sauce. Use whole-grain muffins.

BROCCOLI NUT CASSEROLE

In the Beginning

1 cup broccoli, cut in medium pieces; 1 cup diced tomatoes; ½ cup diced almonds; 1 cup plain yogurt; ¾ cup grated cheese.

Mix all together, except for cheese. Sprinkle cheese on top. Bake in 350° oven, 20 minutes or until broccoli is cooked and cheese is brown and melted. *Serves 4 to 6.*

On Your Way

Use raw natural cheeses. Sprinkle with sesame seeds. Use homemade yogurt.

Top of the Line

Use raw natural cheeses. Sprinkle with sesame seeds. Use homemade yogurt. Serve on bed of brown rice or millet.

LIVER SLIVERS

In the Beginning

½ pound liver; ½ onion, sliced thin; butter or oil for pan; 1 apple, sliced thin.

Place liver in freezer 10 minutes to facilitate cutting process. Slice liver into thin, spaghetti-sized strands. Simmer onions in butter or oil. Add liver and apple slices. Stir-fry quickly, moving pieces about while cooking. Do not overcook. This is a fast process.

On Your Way

Garnish with sprouts.

Top of the Line

Garnish with sprouts. Serve with whole grain bread for fiber and serve with lightly steamed vegetables for added nutrients (and more fiber!)

Luscious Liquids

Cola drinks, soda pop, sugared fruit drinks . . . flush them down the drain. Careful! Some of them may even corrode the pipes. Here are a few choice delicious and nourishing drinks that can really quench your children's thirst.

LIGHT ORANGE FROTH (for the non-breakfast eater)

In the Beginning

1 glass orange juice; 1 raw egg; 1 teaspoon honey-sweetened vanilla ice cream.
    Whip and serve cold.

On Your Way

Eliminate ice cream. Use fresh fruit (pineapple, bananas, peaches).

Top of the Line

Encourage "no snacking" after dinner for the breakfast non-eater. This will surely increase morning appetites. Nothing can substitute for a breakfast which includes a fiber food (whole-grain cereal).

THIRST QUENCHER

In the Beginning

½ cup apple juice; ½ cup sparkling water; pinch of ginger powder.
    Blend.

On Your Way

Use good-quality mineral water instead of sparkling water.

Top of the Line

Use good-quality mineral water instead of sparkling water. Use freshly crushed ginger.

YOGURT SHAKE

In the Beginning

1 cup plain yogurt; 1 cup sliced strawberries; 1 large banana, cut up; 1 cup milk.

Combine in blender. Blend a few seconds until smooth.

On Your Way

Use fresh strawberries or other fresh fruit.

Top of the Line

Use 2 cups yogurt and no milk. Use only fresh fruit.

BANANA SHAKE

In the Beginning

¾ glass milk; 1 raw egg; ½ ripe banana; dash vanilla.

Whip and serve cold. Substitute or add strawberries, canteloupe, peaches, pineapple, or peanut butter.

On Your Way

Use raw certified whole milk.

Top of the Line

Use nut milk instead of regular milk. (See recipe in *Substitute* section.)

The Side Dish

Don't sideline the side dishes. They may provide the missing link to add zest, fiber, or nutrients to round out a meal.

TOFU MOCK COTTAGE CHEESE

In the Beginning

½ pound soft tofu; ¼ cup fresh parsley, finely chopped; ¼ cup fresh scallions, minced; ¼ cup mayonnaise; ½ teaspoon minced garlic; 1 tablespoon cider vinegar.

Let tofu drain in colander while cutting vegetables. Mash tofu into cottage-cheese texture. Combine all other ingredients with tofu; blend until creamy. Chill before serving.

On Your Way

Use sugar-free and additive-free mayonnaise.

Top of the Line

Use sugar-free mayonnaise, without additives. Serve with raw vegetable sticks.

CARROT, CABBAGE, AND RAISIN SALAD

In the Beginning

1 cup finely shredded cabbage; 3 cups grated carrots; ½ cup raisins; ½ cup mayonnaise; ½ teaspoon sea salt; 1 teaspoon raw honey; 2 teaspoons lemon juice.

Mix vegetables and raisins. Mix mayonnaise, salt, honey and lemon juice. Stir all together well.

On Your Way

Use homemade mayonnaise. Eliminate salt and honey.

Top of the Line

Eliminate salt and honey. Use oil-free salad dressing (see *Dressing It Up* section). Add sesame seeds.

POTATO SALAD

In the Beginning

4 large potatoes; 4 hard-cooked eggs; 1 chopped onion; ½ cup celery; 2 tablespoons diced green or red pepper; 2 tablespoons chopped chives; 1 scallion chopped with green top; 1 tablespoon prepared mustard; ½ cup mayonnaise; 2 tablespoons parsley.

Cut potatoes into bits; slice eggs; mix with onion, celery, pepper, chives, scallion and mustard. Add mayonnaise. Garnish with parsley.

On Your Way

Use ¼ cup sugar-free and additive-free mayonnaise and ¼ cup yogurt.

Top of the Line

Use ¼ cup homemade mayonnaise and ¼ cup homemade yogurt. Serve on dark, leafy greens.

Company's Coming

Whether the guests are your children's peers or yours, they'll never suspect that the gourmet food is good for them! And your family will love the leftovers.

BROCCOLI QUICHE

In the Beginning

2 cups chopped broccoli, lightly steamed; 2 beaten eggs; 1 cup milk; 1 cup grated cheese; 1 tablespoon fine, dry whole wheat breadcrumbs; pinch nutmeg; 2 cups cooked brown rice.

Place broccoli in bowl and add all ingredients except rice. Press rice into 9" buttered pie dish. (The rice serves as crust.) Pour mixture into crust. Bake 25 minutes or until "set," at 350°.

On Your Way

Use raw certified whole milk and natural raw cheese.

Top of the Line

Use raw certified whole milk and cheese, and raw broccoli instead of steamed broccoli.

STEAMED CHICKEN

In the Beginning

1 small chicken; 2 cloves garlic, minced; ½ teaspoon paprika; ½ teaspoon oregano.

Place chicken in steamer basket over an inch or two of water. Bring to boil. Steam on low heat for 30 minutes, covered. Remove chicken, cut into eighths. Dust with oregano; sprinkle with garlic and paprika. Place under broiler and broil until golden brown.

On Your Way

Serve with lightly steamed vegetables and whole grain (such as brown rice).

Top of the Line

Use small amount of chicken to embellish large amount of whole grains with diced raw vegetables.

MEATBALLS AND SPAGHETTI (REAL AND "MOCK")

In the Beginning

1 pound ground beef; 1 medium onion, chopped; 1 teaspoon sea salt; 1 tablespoon bread crumbs; 1 tablespoon oil; 2 cups tomato sauce; 1 cup water; 1 pound spaghetti.

Mix meat with ½ of onion. Add salt and bread crumbs. Form into meatballs; brown in oil. Add tomato sauce, water and rest of onion. Simmer for ½ hour. Cook spaghetti according to package directions. When done, add meatballs and sauce.

On Your Way

Use ½ teaspoon salt instead of 1 teaspoon salt. Use 1 cup tomato sauce and 1 cup fresh tomatoes, mashed. Use whole-wheat bread crumbs. Use Jerusalem artichoke or whole wheat spaghetti. Use vegetable stock in place of water. Add ½ pint mushrooms.

Top of the Line

1 16-ounce package tofu; 1 clove minced garlic; 2 tablespoons minced parsley; 1 heaping teaspoon oregano; ½ cup firmly packed minced onion; 2 eggs; ¾ cup whole-wheat bread crumbs (to create complete protein); enough oil for frying; 1 pound buckwheat noodles or whole-wheat noodles; 1 quart natural spaghetti sauce; ½ pound grated Mozzarella cheese.

Drain tofu in colander. Crumble and mash until tofu is creamy.

This is necessary for flexibility in forming "meat" balls. Add garlic, parsley (fresh will have more taste), oregano (use dried for more pungency here), and onions. Break eggs into mixture to hold it together. Mix. Add bread crumbs. Roll into balls (1 heaping tablespoon for each ball). Makes 34 balls. Pour oil into pan and heat. Add tofu balls. Unlike meatballs, you can't put these tofu balls into hot sauce and mix: they will fall apart. Brown on medium heat.

Secret: Use 2 teaspoons to turn as the balls brown. A spatula will break them apart. This is more delicate than meat. Put a little sauce aside, and dump rest (cold) on balls. Bake at 350° until sauce starts to boil. Keep warm until ready to serve.

To prepare for serving, place balls on noodles with rest of sauce on top. Sprinkle cheese on top of sauce. Place under broiler a few minutes and serve as a casserole. It is super delicious. If you tell your family these are Swedish meatballs, they will believe you because Swedish meatballs are mellow, as these are. The association of spaghetti sauce and meat helps too! Enjoy!

TOFU VEGETABLE KEBABS

In the Beginning

2 tablespoons lemon juice; ¼ cup oil; 2 cloves garlic, crushed; ⅛ teaspoon pepper; 3 tablespoons tamari; ½ teaspoon paprika; 1 pound firm tofu; 2 firm tomatoes; 1 large onion; 2 green peppers; 8 large mushrooms.

Drain and slice tofu into 1-inch cubes. Mix first six ingredients and place tofu in the mixture for 1 hour. Preheat broiler. Cut vegetables into large chunks to fit skewers. Alternate vegetable and tofu on skewers. Place filled skewers on cookie sheets; baste well with marinade. Broil 5 to 10 minutes, turning and basting once. *Serves 4 (2 skewers each).*

On Your Way

Use 1½ tablespoons tamari in marinade sauce.

Top of the Line

Use 1½ tablespoons tamari in marinade sauce. Sprinkle sesame seeds on kebabs before broiling.

MOCK CHOPPED LIVER

In the Beginning

1 pound fresh string beans; boiling water; 3 tablespoons oil; 2 large onions, finely chopped; 1 stalk celery, chopped; ¼ cup walnuts, chopped; 3 hard-cooked eggs; 1 teaspoon chopped olives.

Cook string beans in boiling water until tender. Drain beans (save liquid for use in soup); set aside. Heat oil in skillet. Sauté onions until tender. Add celery. Cook 2 minutes longer. Chop beans, onion mixture, walnuts, and eggs. Add olives. *Serves 4.*

On Your Way

Use homemade mayonnaise in place of oil. Lightly steam string beans and celery instead of boiling.

Top of the Line

Use homemade mayonnaise in place of oil. Use raw string beans and celery instead of cooked. Serve with other raw vegetables to upgrade fiber and nutrients.

ENCHANTING CHAPATIS

In the Beginning

2 cups whole-wheat flour; ¼ teaspoon salt; ¾ cup water.

Put flour and salt in bowl. Make well in center; pour in half the water. Mix water into flour with hands to form dough. (If too dry, add more water.) Shape dough into ball. Knead dough on floured surface 10 to 15 minutes (children love to do this), or until smooth. Place damp cloth over dough; set aside 30 minutes. Knead again 5 minutes. Divide into 12 pieces, shaping each one into ball. Flatten balls slightly; roll again on floured surface into 5-inch rounds.

Heat lightly greased griddle or heavy pan. Cook rounds, one at a time on griddle, turning with fingertips. Cook only about 2 minutes, or until bubbles appear on top. Turn, and cook another minute or so, turning as chapati cooks, until brown spots appear on underside.

Use slotted spatula to remove from pan. Hold in open flame until bread puffs. For electric stoves: press bread firmly onto griddle with paper toweling. Chapati will puff when released.

On Your Way

Add 2 tablespoons plain homemade yogurt to flour before adding first quantity of water. Use ⅛ teaspoon salt.

Top of the Line

Eliminate salt. Use freshly stone-ground flour.

AMBROSIA

In the Beginning

½ cup yogurt; ½ cup sour cream; ½ cup cream cheese; ¼ cup unsweet-ened pineapple pieces; ¼ cup unsweetened coconut shreds; ½ cup chopped nuts.

Combine equal parts of sour cream, yogurt, and cream cheese. Mix with pineapple and coconut. Top with nuts.

On Your Way

Use ¾ cup yogurt and ¼ cup sour cream.

Top of the Line

Use ¾ cup yogurt and ¼ cup sour cream; additive-free cream cheese (homemade or purchased at natural food store); fresh pineapple; nuts freshly cracked.

Dressing It Up

Dress it but don't destroy it! Do-it-yourself embellishments en-hance the flavor without the need to post danger signs for stale and rancid oil.

FRESH TOMATO SAUCE

In the Beginning

½ onion, chopped; 1 clove garlic, minced; 2 tablespoons oil; 1 small carrot, grated; 2 tablespoons green pepper, chopped; 1 bay leaf; 1 tea-

spoon oregano; ½ teaspoon thyme; ¼ teaspoon basil; 2 tablespoons fresh parsley, chopped; 2 cups tomatoes, fresh; 1 6-ounce can tomato paste; ½ teaspoon sea salt; ⅛ teaspoon pepper.

Sauté onion and garlic in oil until onion is soft. Add carrot, green pepper, bay leaf, herbs. Stir well. Add tomatoes, tomato paste, seasonings. Simmer 30 minutes. Remove bay leaf. MAKES 2 CUPS.

On Your Way

Use homemade tomato paste.

Top of the Line

Use homemade tomato paste. Eliminate salt. Use unrefined oil.

TOMATO PASTE

In the Beginning

4 tomatoes; ¼ teaspoon salt.

Peel tomatoes after blanching in hot water. Run through strainer. Pour into heavy skillet. Cook slowly over low heat until liquid has boiled off. Takes about 1½ hours for tomatoes to thicken. Stir occasionally while simmering.

On Your Way

Eliminate salt.

Top of the Line

Eliminate salt. Do not peel tomatoes. Mash with fork before simmering.

REAL MAYONNAISE

In the Beginning

1 egg; 2 tablespoons lemon juice or vinegar; 1 cup oil; ½ to 1 teaspoon dry mustard; ¾ teaspoon sea salt; ¼ teaspoon white pepper.

Combine egg, lemon juice, ¼ cup oil, dry mustard, salt and pepper in electric blender. Cover; blend at low speed until mixed. Increase to high speed; uncover or remove center cap. Add remaining oil in thin, slow steady stream. Blend until all oil is added and mayonnaise is smooth and creamy. It may be necessary to turn motor off and stir occasionally. Replace cover before turning motor back on. Keep mayonnaise refrigerated. Use within a week.

On Your Way

Eliminate salt. Use fertile egg. Use freshly squeezed lemon juice.

Top of the Line

Eliminate salt. Use fertile egg. Use freshly squeezed lemon juice. Use unrefined oil.

TOFU-SESAME DRESSING

In the Beginning

1 cup tofu; 1 cup water; 2 tablespoons tamari; ¼ cup tahini sesame butter (ground sesame seeds); 1 tablespoon chopped parsley; 2 to 3 cloves garlic; ½ cup lemon juice.
Blend all ingredients.

On Your Way

Use only 1 tablespoon tamari.

Top of the Line

Use only 1 tablespoon tamari. Add 1 teaspoon kelp.

SUNFLOWER/YOGURT DRESSING

In the Beginning

1 cup sunflower seeds; 1 cup plain yogurt; 2 tablespoons chopped onions; 2 tablespoons chopped celery; 1 tablespoon dill.
Blend all ingredients.

On Your Way

Use homemade, whole-milk yogurt. Add chopped cucumbers.

Top of the Line

Use homemade, whole raw milk yogurt. Add chopped cucumbers. Add 1 tablespoon chopped alfalfa sprouts.

TACO DRESSING

In the Beginning

2 mashed avocados; ½ teaspoon tamari; ½ teaspoon lemon juice; ¼ teaspoon garlic powder. Combine.

On Your Way

Use 1 clove crushed garlic instead of powdered garlic.

Top of the Line

Use 1 clove crushed garlic instead of powdered garlic. Reduce tamari to ¼ teaspoon.

FRUIT CREAM

In the Beginning

1 pound medium tofu; 1 cup crushed pineapple (including juice); 2 heaping tablespoons unsweetened coconut; 1 tablespoon lemon juice; ¼ cup honey; 1 banana (optional).

With blender set on low, place pineapple in blender. Next, add coconut, then lemon juice, next honey, and then banana. Blend until smooth. Now add tofu, ¼ pound at a time. Stir with wooden spoon as mixture blends (cover off). Takes 5 full minutes. Stir only ½-inch into one corner to create a current, which will keep mixture moving. When finished, fruit cream will have consistency of creamy pudding. Serve over fruit.

On Your Way

Eliminate honey.

Top of the Line

Eliminate honey. Use freshly grated coconut, freshly cut pineapple and freshly squeezed lemon.

APPLE SYRUP

In the Beginning

2 tablespoons butter; 2 tablespoons whole-wheat flour; 3 cups apple juice, boiled down to 1½ cups.

Melt butter on low heat. Stir in flour. Gradually add boiled down apple juice, stirring constantly. Raise heat until mixture almost simmers, but do not allow it to boil. Cook, stirring constantly until sauce thickens (about 5 minutes). This sauce is good on pancakes or spooned over plain cake.

On Your Way

Use freshly expressed homemade apple juice.

Top of the Line

Use raw, unsalted butter.
Use freshly (stone) ground flour.
Use freshly expressed homemade apple juice.

The Pie and Cake Bake

Even newborn babies show a definite craving for sweets (they pay little attention to salty or bitter flavor). Sweets should not be emphasized. These recipes are for transitional lifestyle changes and special occasions.[5]

FOR YOUR CRUST

In the Beginning

2 cups whole-wheat flour, sifted; ⅔ cup softened butter; ¼ cup ice water; 1 tablespoon lemon juice; ½ teaspoon cinnamon.
Mix flour in bowl. Use fork or pastry blender to cut butter into flour until mixture is in small bits. Mix ice water and lemon juice. Add ice water and lemon juice to first mixture, 1 tablespoon at a time. Divide mixture in half and roll in between 2 pieces of waxed paper to about ⅛-inch thickness. Bake crust for about 15 minutes at 400°.

On Your Way

Use unsalted butter made from raw milk.

Top of the Line

Use unsalted butter made from raw milk. Grind wheatberries just prior to preparing crust.

GRANOLA PIE

In the Beginning

1⅓ cups granola; ¼ cup softened butter; 8 tart apples; 1 tablespoon cinnamon; ¼ cup softened butter; ½ cup water.

Mix granola and ¼ cup butter; press into 9-inch pie plate. Bake at 350° 6 to 8 minutes. Cool; set aside. Peel apples; slice into buttered casserole. Top with softened butter (¼ cup) and cinnamon. Pour water over apples. Bake at 375° for 45 minutes. Scoop mixture into pie crust. Top with chopped nuts, and place under broiler just a few minutes.

On Your Way

Use unsalted butter made from raw milk.

Top of the Line

Use unsalted butter made from raw milk. Use unsprayed apples and pure spring water.

CARROT CAKE

In the Beginning

10 cups carrots, shredded; 3 cups whole-wheat flour; ½ cup each raisins, dried pineapple, apricots, sunflower seeds, walnuts; 1 teaspoon cinnamon; ½ teaspoon each of nutmeg, coriander, ginger; 1 cup water; 2 eggs (optional).

Mix dry ingredients together. Mix wet ingredients in separate bowl. Mix both together. Place in greased pan. Bake at 350° for 50 minutes or until done.

On Your Way

Use organically grown carrots. Eliminate dried pineapple.

Top of the Line

Use organically grown carrots. Eliminate dried pineapple. Use freshly cracked nuts, spring water, fertile eggs, and stone-ground flour (freshly ground).

CHOCOLATE MOUSSE

In the Beginning

¼ *cup granola; 2 tablespoons butter; 2 squares chocolate; 2 pounds medium tofu (firm tofu won't cream up like sour cream, which is consistency needed);° 2 bananas; ½ cup honey; ½ teaspoon cinnamon; 1 tablespoon real vanilla.*

Grease spring-pan with butter. Blend granola to fine powder. Coat pan with powdered granola (thickly). Melt butter into chocolate in separate pan. Mix all other ingredients into chocolate mix and pour into spring pan. Bake at 350° for 1 hour. Mixture will pull away from sides. Once it cools, it firms again, so don't cook until it cracks (as you would cheesecake). Optional: garnish with whipped cream, more granola, or coconut.

°*Note:* Medium tofu is a good substitute for milk, cream, sour cream, or eggs. Firm tofu takes the place of chicken, beef, or fish. Since firm tofu has more protein, it is a better protein alternative.

On Your Way

Use 2 squares carob instead of chocolate. Add 1 pint yogurt.

Top of the Line

Use 2 squares carob instead of chocolate. Add 1 pint yogurt. Eliminate honey.

The Cookie Crunch

What nostalgic thoughts do you conjure up when you think of the cookies of your childhood? Is it a round cookie with a raisin in the center? Is it getting your portion of dough with which you could shape any form? We hope it's not boxes of Nabisco on the cupboard shelf! A fast-food chain is currently trying to create nostalgia for junk food by suggesting that you take your child to their restaurant whenever there's something special to celebrate. We repeat our philosophy that happy occasions can be associated with *good* food—such as home-baked, delicious (and healthful) cookies!

PEANUT BUTTER COOKIES

In the Beginning

⅓ cup peanut oil; ½ cup raw honey; ⅔ cup noncommercial peanut butter; 1 well-beaten egg; 1½ cups whole-wheat flour, sifted; 1 teaspoon cinnamon.

Beat oil and honey well. Add egg and peanut butter; beat. Add flour; mix. Drop by teaspoonful on oiled cookie sheet. Bake 7 to 10 minutes, watching carefully. Don't overbake. Your children will love making these easy-to-prepare cookies.

On Your Way

Use unrefined oil and homemade peanut butter.

Top of the Line

Use unrefined oil and homemade peanut butter. Cut honey to ¼ cup. Use freshly stone-ground flour.

OATMEAL-BANANA COOKIES

In the Beginning

2 cups oat flakes; 2 cups whole-wheat pastry flour; ¾ cup oil; ¾ cup chopped nuts; ¾ cup raisins; 2 bananas, mashed; 1 cup apple juice.

Mix flakes and flour. Stir in oil. Add remaining ingredients. Add a little flour if necessary to stiffen. Drop onto oiled cookie sheet; bake about 30 minutes at 350°. Makes 4 dozen. (This recipe uses no honey!)

On Your Way

Soak raisins several hours before baking. Use freshly shelled nuts.

Top of the Line

Soak raisins several hours before baking. Use freshly shelled nuts. Use unrefined oil and freshly expressed apple juice.

Fun Foods

The refrigerator is brimming over with food. Complex carbohydrates have taken over. The children open the door, and after a thirty-second survey, they comment, "THERE'S NOTHING TO EAT." Fun foods are helpful during the kitchen-transition stage.

LINDA'S MINI MARVELS

In the Beginning

3 eggs, well beaten; 1 cup chopped walnuts; 8 ounces chopped dates or raisins.

Mix everything together. Spoon into greased and floured *tiny* muffin tins. Bake at 350°, 20 minutes. Makes 24 small taste treats. Note: you must use mini-tins. This recipe is especially helpful for the wheat-sensitive.

On Your Way

Soak raisins prior to use. Use fresh dates.

Top of the Line

Soak raisins prior to use. Use fresh dates. Use freshly cracked, untreated walnuts. Use fertile eggs.

NUTTY CHEWS

In the Beginning

½ cup wheat sprouts; ½ cup almonds or other nuts; ½ cup raisins; ⅛ teaspoon sea salt.

Grind all ingredients together. Shape into small balls. Sprouts are sweetest when short, about ¼ inch long, including the grain. MAKES 1 DOZEN.

On Your Way

Soak raisins prior to use. Eliminate salt.

Top of the Line

Soak raisins prior to use. Eliminate salt. Use freshly cracked nuts, untreated.

PEANUT BUTTER-BANANA POPS

In the Beginning

1 cup milk; 1 ripe banana, cut into chunks; ½ cup creamy peanut butter; ½ teaspoon vanilla extract; chopped nuts.

Combine milk and banana in blender and purée until smooth. Add peanut butter and vanilla. Blend well. Pour into freezer molds. Sprinkle with chopped nuts, seal, and freeze until very firm. Unmold and serve immediately. Roll in chopped nuts.

On Your Way

Use raw milk (certified); freshly cracked, untreated nuts.

Top of the Line

Use raw milk (certified); freshly cracked, untreated nuts, home-made peanut butter, and pure vanilla extract.

CHEESE BALL

In the Beginning

2 eight-ounce packages cream cheese; 1 eight-ounce can crushed, unsweetened pineapple, drained; 2 cups chopped toasted pecans; ¼ cup finely chopped onion; ¼ cup finely chopped green pepper.

Combine cheese, pineapple, 1 cup pecans, onion, pepper. Form into 1 large or 2 small balls. Roll in remaining pecans. Refrigerate overnight.

On Your Way

Use fresh pineapple. Use additive-free cream cheese.

Top of the Line

Use fresh pineapple. Use additive-free cheese. Use untoasted pecans, freshly hulled.

ALMOND CRUNCH CHEWIES

In the Beginning

⅓ cup butter; ¼ cup honey; ¾ cup slivered almonds.

Melt butter in skillet; stir honey into butter. Add almonds. Cook at medium temperature. Stir while cooking. Takes about 6 to 8 minutes for mixture to turn golden-brown. Spread in prepared pan while mixture is still hot. Use oiled or buttered sharp knife to cut into squares while hot. After cooling, place in refrigerator in covered container.

On Your Way

Use raw milk butter.

Top of the Line

Use raw milk butter, unfiltered raw honey and freshly hulled, untreated almonds.

RASPBERRY SURPRISE

In the Beginning

2 eight-ounce cakes tofu; 1½ teaspoons vanilla; 2 tablespoons lemon juice; 1 ten-ounce package frozen raspberries; 1 ripe, mashed banana; ½ cup honey; dash salt.

Mix tofu, vanilla and lemon juice. Drain juice from raspberries, and add to mixture with balance of ingredients. Blend all in mixer at high speed. Chill. *Serves 6.*

On Your Way

Eliminate salt. Use ¼ cup honey instead of ½ cup.

Top of the Line

Eliminate salt and honey. Use fresh raspberries. Use pure vanilla.

PINEAPPLE YOGURT FREEZE

In the Beginning

1 cup plain yogurt; 1 cup crushed pineapple, unsweetened.

Place yogurt in freezer tray and freeze to mush. Remove. Add crushed pineapple and juice. Return to freezer. Freeze to soft mush. Place in mixing bowl; mix well. Return to tray. Freeze until solid. For variety, add strawberries, diced peaches, or unsweetened grape juice to yogurt. *Serves 4.*

On Your Way

Use homemade yogurt.

Top of the Line

Use homemade yogurt. Use fresh pineapple.

SWEET POTATO CANDY

In the Beginning

2 large baked sweet potatoes (about 1 pound); 2 ripe bananas; 1 egg yolk, beaten; 1 teaspoon lemon juice; 1 teaspoon allspice; ½ cup wheat germ; 1 egg white, beaten; ½ cup ground walnuts; oil or butter.

Peel and mash potatoes with banana, egg yolk, lemon juice and allspice. Refrigerate until thoroughly chilled and then form into balls. Roll in wheat germ and refrigerate again for ½ hour. Roll in egg whites and nuts. Lightly fry until golden-brown.

On Your Way

Use fertile eggs and freshly squeezed lemon juice.

Top of the Line

Use fertile eggs and freshly squeezed lemon juice. Replace wheat germ with whole-wheat bread crumbs or ground, sprouted wheatberries.

APRICOT LEATHER

In the Beginning

4 cups boiling water; 4 cups dried apricots; 4 tablespoons honey.

Pour water over apricots. Let sit 24 hours. Blend in blender. Add honey. Prepare cookie sheet with oiled wax paper. Spread apricot mixture thinly and evenly. Let dry 2 days. Peel off and wrap in plastic wrap. Cut in 1-inch pieces.

On Your Way

Use unsulfured apricots, soaked for several hours. Use 2 tablespoons honey.

Top of the Line

Use unsulfured apricots, soaked for several hours. Use 1 tablespoon honey. Use spring water.

FRUIT CREAM DESSERT

In the Beginning

Chill or freeze any pieces of fresh fruit (bananas, berries, etc.). Blend. Pour into ice cube trays. Freeze. Blend again. Freeze again. Top with yogurt, nuts, coconut, mashed pineapple.

On Your Way

Use unsprayed fruit.

Top of the Line

Use unsprayed fruit, homemade yogurt, freshly hulled, untreated nuts, freshly grated coconut.

THE ZUCKER TWINS' PIZZA—BOTTOM PART

In the Beginning

1½ tablespoons dry baking yeast; 1¼ cups warm water; 1 teaspoon honey; ¼ cup olive oil; 1 teaspoon oregano; 1 teaspoon basil; 2¾ cups whole-wheat flour.
Dissolve yeast in water and honey. Mix with oil, herbs and flour. Let rise in bowl in warm place until volume doubles (about 1½ hours). Punch down. Knead again for a few minutes so dough will handle easily. Divide dough in half. Stretch; roll out to ⅛″ thickness. Place a little flour in 2 pans. Place pizza dough in pans. Pinch up edges.

On Your Way

Use spring water and ½ teaspoon honey.

Top of the Line

Use spring water and ½ teaspoon honey. Add ½ teaspoon kelp. Use freshly stone-ground flour.

TOPPING FOR PIZZA

In the Beginning

¾ cup tomato sauce; ¼ cup grated mozzarella cheese; grated Parmesan cheese.

Mix all and bake 10 to 15 minutes at 450°. Optional toppings: green pepper, garlic, avocado, sunflower seeds, etc. Makes 2 pizzas.

On Your Way

Use homemade tomato sauce.

Top of the Line

Use homemade tomato sauce. Use additive-free cheeses made from whole raw milk.

SESAME CRISP CRACKERS

In the Beginning

1 cup oat flour; ¾ cup soy flour; ¼ cup sesame seeds; ¼ cup oil; ½ cup water; ¾ teaspoon salt.

Combine oat and soy flour, sesame seeds and salt. Add oil. Blend. Mix to pie dough consistency. Roll out dough to ⅛ inch thickness on oiled cookie sheets. Cut out with cookie cutters (let the kids do it) or with crinkled pie cutter. Bake in preheated oven until crackers are brown (about 15 minutes).

On Your Way

Eliminate salt.

Top of the Line

Eliminate salt. Use freshly stone-ground flour.

MATTHEW'S PUDDING AND KRISTA'S VARIATION

In the Beginning

2 packets tofu (or 2 big chunks—exact amounts not important); 1 ripe or 2 medium-ripe bananas; 2 seedless oranges; nutmeg and cinnamon to taste; ¼ cup apple juice; 4 ice cubes.

Blend tofu, bananas, oranges, and spices. Add ice cubes one at a time. Add just enough apple juice to smooth (this will prevent tofu from becoming grainy). Blend to consistency of shake (excuse the expression) and pour into custard cups.

Optional additions: brown rice, raisins, nuts, seeds, coconut, sprouted wheatberries, strawberries, papaya, peaches. Mix any of these additions through pudding. *Krista's variation:* cut down on banana and orange and add carob.

On Your Way

Use untreated, organic oranges.

Top of the Line

Use untreated, organic oranges. Use freshly squeezed apple juice.

Lunchbox Logic

We used to think that if the dietary protein sources were derived primarily from fish, meat, milk, eggs or cheese, we would be fostering the best of health. After all, aren't these foods considered to be of high biological value? Ah, but where's the zinc? If you are a luncheon-meat family, take heed.

One mother, frustrated because of the difficulties of her food-life-style changes, said, "I think I'll turn the children loose and let them eat what they catch." Hopefully, our suggestions for lunch and brown-bagging will prevent fumbling and put the ball in your court.

Lunchbox Logic Generalities

☆ *Variety of foods:* No single food supplies all the essential nutrients in amounts needed. The greater the variety in a single lunch box, the less chance of nutritional deficiency. The diversity will also reduce the likelihood of exposure to excessive amounts of specific contaminants which may be found in any single food item. *Vary the food in the lunchbox.*

☆ *Rotation of foods:* Try not to repeat identical foods day after day.

(Peanut butter and jelly sandwiches?) Repetition of foods and consumption of large quantities of the same food encourages allergy. *Rotate the food in the lunchbox.*

☆ *Do-it-yourself arrangement:* Wrap all the makings of a sandwich
separately (use sectioned plastic containers with tight lid), and let the
children assemble the lunch at school. For example, pack bread,
mayonnaise, sliced chicken, lettuce, cucumbers, individually. *Pack the
makings of the lunch separately in the lunchbox.*

☆ *Carnival preparations:* Use animal cookie cutters on whole-grain
bread to prepare nut-butter sandwiches in delightful shapes. Roll
shredded cheese, chopped chicken, and chopped nuts into balls. *Festive foods should enter the lunchbox from time to time.*

☆ *Wholistic food fare:* On occasion, pack a whole apple, a large
chunk of bread (broken from an unsliced loaf), a wedge of cheese, nuts
in the shell and a nutcracker (or peanuts in the shell for the younger
set), and green peas in their pods. *Use natural foods in their natural
architecture.*

☆ *Limitation of fruits:* Children have small stomach capacities.
Therefore, what they eat should be nutrient-dense. Fruit does *not* fit
this category. Fruit is low in fiber (compared to whole grains and
bread), and the fact that fruit contains simple sugars lowers its rating
on our *one to ten* scale. Unlike a seed, a nut or a grain, fruit does *not*
provide nourishment for its seed.[6] *Limit the fruit in the lunchbox.*

☆ *Palate-pleaser condiments:* To spruce up bland mixtures, use prepared mustard, fresh chives, horseradish, chili sauce, grated Parmesan
cheese, chopped olives, fresh oregano, etc. *Add tasty seasonings.*

☆ *Value of seeds:* Seeds are dormant plants, chock full of nutrients,
waiting for the opportune time to grow. They are high in both protein
and fat (the good-guy type of fat).[7] *Include nuts, seeds, and legumes in
the lunchbox.*

☆ *Attractive presentation:* The precise cutting and cooking of vegetables to retain shape, color, texture and crispness is more than the
fancy of the Oriental chef. Our Far Eastern friends know the importance of eye appeal. Carrots, peppers, zucchini, cucumbers, squash,
celery, and sweet potato are irresistible when cut into noodle-sized
strips. *Include raw vegetables cut in small, attractive bits in the
lunchbox.*

☆ *Offerings with love:* Good food served with love! What a combination! As part of the trimmings, insert little notes which read, "I love you." "You are so special." "Looking forward to 3:00 P.M." "Looking forward to 6:00 P.M." "Let's plan a surprise for Daddy tonight." "Let's shop for Mom's birthday on Saturday." "Just a reminder—only 3 weeks until we go fishing." "Grandma says you should call her tonight; she misses you." "Have a happy day." "I had fun preparing your lunch; enjoy it." "Isn't Ms. (or Mr.) So-and-So (the teacher) lucky? She (or he) can be with you all day." *Include TLC in the lunchbox.*

☆ *Salad combinations:* Don't lock yourself into sandwiches. Expose the children to salads. Throw a pair of chopsticks into the lunchbox (after you have taught your children how to use them). *Include salads in the lunchbox.*

Lunchbox Logic Specifics

Peanut butter mixtures:
1. ½ cup peanut butter, 1 teaspoon lemon juice, 1 teaspoon unsweetened coconut, 1 teaspoon sunflower seeds, 1 teaspoon sesame seeds, 3 chopped dates, 2 tablespoons shredded apple.
2. Add any one of the following to peanut butter:
   Grated raw carrot
   Alfalfa sprouts
   Peach and/or banana slices
   Sliced apples and/or sliced grapes

To prevent roof-of-mouth sticking, add a few drops of orange juice to peanut butter mixtures. And of course, use homemade or unsweetened, unhydrogenated peanut butter. Try almond, cashew, sesame, and sunflower butters. Combine nut butters.

Fill whole wheat pita pouches with:
   Any combination of salads
   Yogurt with bits of raw broccoli and sprouts
   Shredded carrot, egg and avocado slices
   Cream cheese and homemade granola
   Grated carrots, eggs and chopped pecans
   Mashed baked beans with onion and grated cheese

    Cream cheese, pineapple and nuts
    Salmon with chopped cucumbers
    Chicken and apple slices
Roll these fillings in a cabbage leaf instead of bread, or stuff into a green or red pepper.

Steam eggs to hardness by placing in steamer basket over boiling water. Turn heat down, cover pot, and experiment with time (every setup varies). An inexpensive egg puncher will punch a pin-sized hole in the eggs, releasing air, thereby preventing eggs from cracking while cooking. Dye hard-cooked eggs to lend an air of festivity. Use beet juice to color eggs red; grass stains to color green.

Dip grapes and banana slices in coconut, and freeze. To keep frozen in the lunchbox, pack with small can of well-wrapped chemical ice (freezer gel in cans; available in hardware stores).

Scoop out celery sticks, zucchini, squash, cucumber, green peppers. Fill with nut butters, bean paste, grated carrot with cream cheese and raisins, cheddar cheese, with softened butter and garden relish. Top with shredded raw cheese, caraway seeds, or sesame seeds. Place two halves together to close contents.

Add any of the following to plain yogurt: carob, grape juice (unsweetened), vanilla, granola, nuts and seeds, grated raw milk cheese, vegetable bits.

For cold days, cut up fresh vegetables and place in thermos with hot water, herbs, and bouillon seasonings.

These sandwich spreads are delicious on sprouted grain breads:
    Mashed avocado with buckwheat or sunflower lettuce (see Sprouting section)
    Equal amounts of ground sesame seeds and soft butter, with a handful of sprouted lentils

Buy fresh coconuts, and make the process of opening them a family project. Store in refrigerator, and break off pieces to include in lunchboxes.

Sprouting Instructions

Soak one or two tablespoons of seeds or beans in one cup of water overnight. In the morning, pour the water off. (Use this water for your plants—they'll love it! Or save the water as the Hanssens do, as explained in the Epilogue.) Rinse the seeds. Place seeds in glass jar at a slight angle, so that any water will run off. Sprouts like moisture, but not puddles. Rinse the seeds again, two or three times a day. One way to do this is to dump the seeds into a strainer, rinse, and shake by tapping the strainer against the side of the sink. Then replace the seeds in the jar. Or: cover jar with nylon mesh netting, and run rinsing water directly into the jar. The mesh is held in place with a rubberband, so that seeds won't escape when you pour the water off.

It's advisable to start the growing procedure in the dark. However, if you hide the jars in a closet, more than likely you will forget they are there, and you will be unveiling something not unlike Pandora's box a week or more later. So place the jar in a paper bag, and leave on your kitchen counter.

Seeds may be consumed at any stage of sprouting, but harvesting at peak offers the most nutrient value. It has been shown that vitamin C is actually synthesized during germination, and the concentration of some of the B vitamins is also increased during the sprouting process.[8]

Since all seeds vary, it is advisable to experiment, using a good sprouting book as a guide. (See *Book References* in the Appendix.) Alfalfa, mung, and garbanzo beans are excellent sprouts for beginners. Before consuming, leave sprouts in indirect sunlight. This will "green" the leaves, adding chlorophyll.

Suggestions for use of sprouts:

Alfalfa sprouts enhance deviled eggs or any salad

Wheat grains add zest and crunchiness to salads

Soy bean sprouts simmered with fish are super

Lentils in soup add a mild spicy touch

Garbanzos add crispness to salads

Garbanzos are *real* hamburger helpers: equal parts of ground meat and sprouted chick peas slice beautifully for sandwiches when cold

Sprouts, refrigerated, will last up to a week. However, since they are growing in your kitchen, the "farm" couldn't be closer! Harvest as needed. The nutrient value will be at peak that way.

Growing Buckwheat and Sunflower Lettuce

The basic procedure involves soaking seeds overnight, draining the seeds, and spreading them out on a ½-inch base of soil. Seeds should be watered twice a day, and kept in the dark until blades are about 4 inches high. Growth should now continue in the light. Continue watering twice a day. These sprouts are usually ready in about 7 days. Again—a good book that includes detailed instructions is a worthwhile investment. (One such book is *Healthy Children: Nature's Way* by Ann Wigmore.) The reward for this effort is more than an incredible supply of nutrients: These greens are delicious.

Home Dehydration

Making Your Own "Chips"

Believe it or not, you can compete with potato chips. The answer is thinly sliced, dehydrated sweet potato rounds! Let us introduce you to *home dehydration.* Dried *fruit* is common in our culture. Extend the same principle to *vegetables* and *sprouts* for a taste surprise (and nutrition treat).

What to dry? Sweet potatoes, tomatoes, onions, beets, zucchini, green pepper, mushrooms, mung sprouts, wheat sprouts and lentil sprouts. Slice vegetables very, very thin. Thick slices will get moldy. Food processors work best for thin slicing.

Run an extension cord with a 150-watt bulb at the end of it into your oven. Or, if you already have a light bulb in your oven, change the bulb to the designated wattage. Place the food on the oven rack if you cannot secure some plastic or nylon screening for aeration. You can purchase this screening in a hardware or camping store. (Ask for bug netting.) Drying time generally takes between 24 to 36 hours. If your vegie slices dry longer, mold will develop. Slices should not be too thick, nor heat too low.

Although drying does not replace fresh food, it is a way of preserving food and it is a replacement for the common potato chips, pretzels, and other fried, roasted, and sweetened snacks. Drying does retain more nutritional value than toasting, roasting, steaming, baking or frying because the temperatures are so low (approximately 95° to 125°F). If we had young children today, we would master the technique of vegetable drying, and we would keep a supply of these dried goodies on hand at all times. You have a treat in store for your family. You might start with apples—they're the easiest. (See the *Resource* list in the Appendix for commercial dehydrators. This is a worthwhile investment for families with young children.)

Substitutions

It has been stated that when it comes to food, there are no substitutions, only adventures. The following replacement ideas should be of help:

THICKENING AGENTS

Ground toasted pumpkin seeds, nuts, almonds, walnuts, pecans or peanuts; agar-agar sticks or flakes.

MAYONNAISE

Make your own, or dilute commercial mayonnaise with yogurt.

SOY SAUCE

Use tamari diluted with water.

MILK

1) In cooked recipes, use sesame milk. The recipe: 1 cup sesame seeds, 4 cups of water and 1 tablespoon honey. Toast seeds in 300°-oven for

20 minutes. Combine half of the seeds with half of the water and honey in blender; process until seeds are liquefied—only a minute or two. Repeat blending with second half of ingredients. Strain, forcing as much water as possible from soaked seeds. Refrigerate liquid—this is your sesame milk. (Instead of discarding leftover seed pulp, add it to cookie dough.)

2) Soak ½ cup almonds in 2 cups unsweetened apple juice overnight. Grind in blender next day with 1 tablespoon tahini (sesame seed butter) and ½ teaspoon vanilla. Cinnamon and nutmeg may be added.

3) Soak ¼ cup sesame or sunflower seeds and 5 to 8 dates in 2 cups of water overnight. Blend. Consistency should be smooth. Strain. Refrigerate.

Who could say it better than William Wordsworth:
> *Come forth into the light of things.*
> *Let Nature be your teacher.*[9]

Now hear this from the Kamens:
> *The real power of your household*
> *Is in your kitchen.*

EPILOGUE

Diana Hanssen flipped the radio dial with one hand as she reached into the freezer for the evening's dinner with the other. She stopped short as she heard, "We let our children play hookey one day each spring. A child should know the pleasure of staying home when all the other children are in school." "What kind of fairy tale is that?" thought Diana. "Don't those children ever get sick?" Curious, Diana listened for more. And that moment, Diana's life changed. She tells her story.

Second Opinion

—By Diana Hanssen, mother of
Matthew (8) and Krista (6)

Once upon a time we thought that nutrition awareness meant choosing a darker-colored bread at the bakery, and using brown sugar instead of white. As this information changed places with the truth, we journeyed through the land of honey and morning milkshakes, supermarket granola cereal, and milk, milk, and more milk. And oh, yes—there were the health-food-store cookies, plus packaged health food this and that. It didn't work! We still had bronchitis every other week; we still had infections, 105° fevers, and every other kid on the block's hacking cough.

Everything came to a head a few summers ago. Matthew's middle ear was the recipient of any cold or virus that passed through our town. It was soon apparent that Matthew suffered hearing loss in both ears. We made numerous and very expensive trips to an ear specialist, who convinced us that removal of Matthew's adenoids, plus the insertion of "tubes" in his ears, would solve the problem. Briefly, here is the hospital story.

Matthew was admitted to the hospital the day before the operation, and was X-rayed. Because of some "slip" in the process, I was told he had to be re-X-rayed later that day. To pass the time, I calmly prepared Matthew for the events of the next day—the kind of loving, caring TLC that any parent imparts to a child during crisis time. I assured him that the hospital would help in every way it could. This is how the hospital "helped":

1) Dinner was sent to Matthew the night before his scheduled operation. How lucky that I was there to intercept at the door. Dinner consisted of white starchies, inedible, tough, *uncut* meat, and—are you ready?—THE LARGEST PIECE OF CHERRY PIE I EVER SAW. I whipped out my concealed light, body-building provisions (you have to sneak good food into hospitals).

2) There was so much talk, laughter, and racket outside Matthew's door that night, I wondered how any child in the ward could possibly sleep. I elected to stay overnight, and had to sleep on the floor of this fine (expensive) Long Island, New York hospital.

3) Next morning, right on schedule, the nurse arrived to give Matthew his injection. He drowsily kissed me, and I went to the waiting room. The operation was to take place at 9:00 A.M. At 9:04 the waiting room aid tapped me on the shoulder and announced that the operation had been canceled.

Why?

Later, the head nurse explained that there had been a "mixup" and the results of the X-rays (both sets?) had not been sent to the anesthesiologist *prior* to Matthew's arrival in the operating room. Matthew was already primed for the operation when it was discovered that he had a slight spot on his lung, indicating a minor infection. I watched Matthew as he reacted to the preoperation injection. He drooled, he was groggy, he was uncoordinated, and of course he slept most of the day. He had been drugged unnecessarily.

As we scooped him up to take him home, the head nurse told us we could bring him back in one or two weeks (for new X-rays), and they would "try again." Controlling my inner rage, I demanded to see a high hospital official, to whom I recounted the hospital's mistakes. I left the hospital knowing that there had to be a better way.

I share this story for two reasons:

1) If children must be hospitalized, let us be watchful parents. . . . but more important—

2) Let's find *health* before we resort to medicine and/or operations.

The Better Way

I listened more carefully to nutrition information, and happened to hear Betty Kamen, on WMCA Radio in New York, make the comment that milk often causes mucus problems. Dare I take Matthew's milk away? What about calcium? What about protein? What about grandmothers? Vitamins A and D? Desperation said, "Try it."

It's been two and a half years since we gave up milk. In that time, Matthew has had only one short bout with fever, and my daughter Krista has had none. Matthew has no hearing problems, nor does he have tubes, nor did he ever go back for his operation. He is healthier than he has ever been. Our "milk" is a diet of whole, natural foods.

—D.H.

Appendix A

RECOMMENDED READING

GENERAL

Benowicz, Robert J., *Vitamins and You* (New York: Grosset & Dunlap, 1979).

Buchman, Dian Dincin, *Herbal Medicine: The Natural Way to Get Well and Stay Well* (New York: David McKay Co., Inc., 1979).

———, *Water Therapy* (New York: E. P. Dutton, 1979)

Burkitt, Denis, *Eat Right To Stay Healthy and Enjoy Life More* (New York: Arco Publishing, Inc., 1979).

Bland, Jeffrey, *Your Health Under Siege: Using Nutrition to Fight Back* (Brattleboro, VT: The Stephen Greene Press, 1981).

Dufty, William, *Sugar Blues* (Radnor, PA: Chilton Book Company, 1975).

Gruberg, Edward R. and Raymond, Stephen A., *Beyond Cholesterol* (New York: St. Martin's Press, 1981).

Hall, Ross Hume, *Food for Nought: The Decline in Nutrition* (New York: Vintage Books, 1976).

Hunter, Beatrice Trum, *Consumer Beware* (New York: Simon and Schuster, 1971).

———, *The Great Nutrition Robbery* (New York: Charles Scribner's Sons, 1978).

———, *How Safe Is the Food in Your Kitchen?* (New York: Charles Scribner's Sons, 1981).

Kalokerinos, Archie, *Every Second Child* (New Canaan, CT: Keats Publishing, Inc., 1981).

Kinderlehrer, Jane, *Confessions of a Sneaky Organic Cook* (Emmaus, PA: Rodale Press, 1971).

Kirschmann, John D., *Nutrition Almanac* (New York: McGraw-Hill Book Co., 1973).

Mannerberg, Don, and Roth, June, *Aerobic Nutrition* (New York: Hawthorn/Dutton, 1981).

Price, Weston A., *Nutrition and Physical Degeneration* (Santa Monica, CA: The Price-Pottenger Nutrition Foundation, Inc., 1945).

Schauss, Alexander, *Diet, Crime and Delinquency* (Berkeley, CA: Parker House, 1980).

Shannon, Ira L., *Brand Name Guide to Sugar* (Chicago, IL: Nelson-Hall, 1977).

Smith, Lendon, *Feed Your Kids Rights* (New York: McGraw-Hill Book Co., 1979).

The New York Institute for Child Development with Richard J. Walsh, *Treating Your Hyperactive and Learning Disabled Child* (Garden City, N.Y.: Anchor Press/Doubleday, 1979).

Whittlesey, Marietta, *Killer Salt* (New York: Balder Press, 1977).

Wigmore, Ann, *Healthy Children: Nature's Way* (Boston: Hippocrates Health Institute).

Yepsen, Roger B., and the editors of Rodale Press, *Home Food Systems* (Emmaus, PA: Rodale Press, 1981).

COOKBOOKS

Ford, Frank, *The Simpler Life Cookbook* (Fort Worth, TX: Harvest Press, 1974).

Ford, Marjorie Winn, Hillyard, Susan, and Koock, Mary Faulk, *The Deaf Smith Country Cookbook* (New York: Collier Books, 1973).

Kulvinskas, Viktoras, *Sprout for the Love of Everybody* (Wethersfield, CT: OMango D'Press, 1978).

Roth, June, *Cooking for Your Hyperactive Child* (Chicago: Contemporary Books, 1978).

Shurtleff, William, and Aoyagi, Akiko, *The Book of Tofu: Food for Mankind* (Brookline, MA: Autumn Press, Inc., 1975).

Smith, Lendon, *Foods for Healthy Kids* (New York: McGraw-Hill Book Co., 1981).

Whyte, Karen Cross, *The Complete Sprouting Cookbook* (San Francisco: Troubador Press, 1973).

Zucker, Judi and Shari, *Eat Without Meat: Naturally* (Santa Barbara, CA: Woodbridge Press Publ. Co., 1981).

————, *How to Survive Snack Attacks: Naturally* (Santa Barbara, CA: Woodbridge Press Publ. Co., 1979).

PREGNANCY

Kamen, Betty and Kamen, Si, *The Kamen Plan for Total Nutrition During Pregnancy* (E. Norwalk, CT: Appleton-Century-Crofts, 1981).

MAGAZINES

East-West Journal, 17 Station Street, Brookline, MA 02146.

The Health Quarterly, Keats Publishing Co., 27 Pine St., New Canaan, CT 06840.

Let's Live, 444 N. Larchmont Blvd., Los Angeles, CA 90004.

Prevention, Rodale Press, Organic Park, Emmaus, PA 18049.

Public Scrutiny, monthly magazine of the National Health Federation, 212 West Foothill, Monrovia, CA 91016.

Appendix B

PARENT SUPPORT SYSTEMS AND BEHAVIOR MODIFICATION

Check with local schools and telephone directory for any parent-support groups. Parent effectiveness training courses and behavior modification groups can be very helpful while going through the nutrition transitions.

BOOKS

Baruch, Dorothy W., *New Ways in Discipline* (New York: McGraw-Hill, 1949).

Erikson, Eric H., *Identity, Youth and Crisis* (New York: W.W. Norton, 1968).

Ginott, Haim G., *Between Parent and Child* (New York: Macmillan, 1973).

Gordon, Thomas, *Parent Effectiveness Training* (New York: Wyden Books, 1970).

Holt, John, *Escape from Childhood: Freedom and Beyond* (New York: Dell, 1973).

————, *How Children Fail* (New York: Dell, 1982).

————, *How Children Learn* (New York: Dell, 1970).

Mander, Jerry, *Four Arguments for the Elimination of Television* (New York: Morrow-Quill Paperbacks, 1978).

Olsen, Paul, *Sons and Mothers: Why Men Behave As They Do* (New York: M. Evans, 1981).

Pearse, Joseph Chilton, *Magical Child: Rediscovering Nature's Plan for Our Children* (New York: Dutton, 1977).

Piaget, Jean, *The Language and Thought of a Child* (New York: Humanities Press, 1950).

Rogers, Carl, *Freedom to Learn* (Columbus, OH: Charles E. Merrill).

Appendix C

TWELVE DAYS OF CHANGE
(One a Month)

Toby attended a series of nutrition lectures.

On the first day, she discarded all the white bread. On the second day she threw out all the sugar. On the third day she did away with the boxed breakfast cereals. On the fourth day her family got rid of *her!* **Moral:** *Don't make changes too rapidly, unless there is a crisis situation.*

Here's the one-change-a-month plan:

1) Discard nothing. Serve healthful snacks throughout the day. (Cut up raw vegetable strips; fruit; nuts and seeds in the shell, etc.).

2) Serve whole-grain breads. Eliminate the white bread.

3) Eliminate the sugar bowl. Buy fresh pineapple and coconuts and bananas to satisfy the sweet tooth.

4) Eliminate the salt shaker. Use a range of herbs in cooking and in salads.

5) Add small amounts of plain, homemade yogurt to *each* meal.

6) Start sprouting. Add sprouts to *everything.*

7) Serve grain dishes and/or fish as main entrée several times a week.

8) Avoid all red meat, and processed luncheon meats.

9) Throw the can opener away. Use only fresh vegetables (raw or lightly steamed).

10) Use freezer for breads only.

11) Eliminate most milk and milk products (unless of the highest quality and/or fermented).

12) Try vegetable juicing. (You need a juicerator for this one.) Get organic produce if possible, or grow your own.

Have family meetings to discuss the changes. This might avoid or curtail the complaints. Good luck! We hope your children won't be saying, "Must I stay for dinner?"

Appendix D

RESOURCES

FOOD

Organic nuts in the shell
 Jaffe Bros.
 P.O. Box 636
 Valley Center, CA 92082
Herbs and teas
 Meadowbrook Farms
 Wyoming, RI 01898
Organically grown food: bagged and canned
 Arrowhead Mills   *Walnut Acres*
 P.O. Box 866   Penns Creek, PA 17862
 Hereford, TX 79045

 Shiloh Farms
 P.O. Box 97
 Sulphur Springs, AR 72768
Apples
 Kaste's Morningside
 Galesville, WI 54630

ORGANIZATIONS

Feingold Association
1029 Jericho Turnpike
Smithtown, NY 11787
 Volunteer group of parents aimed at helping hyperactive children nationwide.

La Leche League International
9616 Minneapolis Avenue
Franklin Park, IL 60131
  Information and assistance in breastfeeding
National Health Federation
212 Foothill Boulevard
Monrovia, CA 91016
  Excellent health-freedom organization, monthly journal and area
  conventions
New York Institute for Child Development
202 Lexington Avenue
New York, NY 10016
  Treatment for children; nutrition counseling; newsletter, "Reaching Children" (about diet, behavior and learning disabilities).

FILMSTRIPS FOR NUTRITION EDUCATION

Encore Visual Education, Inc.
1235 South Victory Boulevard
Burbank, CA 91502
(213) 843–6515
  Beans, Beans, Beans
  Fruitful Menus
  Grain Cookery
  Vegetarianism: Healthful Eating
  Food: The Choice Is Yours
  The Tofu Experience
  Kitchen With a Mission: Nutrition
  The Seed Sprout Secret
  The Peanut Butter Caper
Bergwall Productions
839 Stewart Ave.
P.O. Box 238
Garden City, NY 11530
(800) 645–3565
  Exploding Nutrition Myths—1
  The Food-Group Foolers

Appendix E

CHANGING THE SCHOOL LUNCH

Resource List

School Lunch Action Guide
> Center for Science in the Public Interest
> 1755 S. Street, N.W.
> Washington, D.C. 20009

Junk Foods Out of School and *A Brown Bag for Your School Child*
> Jane Kinderlehrer
> Rodale Press
> Emmaus, PA 18049

Better Food for Public Places
> Ann Moyer
> Rodale Press
> Emmaus, PA 18049

School Lunch Program
> Lorraine Drexel
> East Aurora Union Free School District
> 430 Main Street
> East Aurora, NY 14052

A Guide for Nutra Lunches and Natural Foods
> Sara Sloan
> Fulton County Schools
> 786 Cleveland Ave., S.W.
> Atlanta, GA 30315

From Classroom to Cafeteria
> Sara Sloan

Fulton County Schools
786 Cleveland Ave., S.W.
Atlanta, GA, 30315
Educational Filmstrips
    See listings in Appendix D

REFERENCES

Chapter 1

1. *Webster's New World Dictionary*, 2nd College ed. (1976), p. 974.

2. Ross Hume Hall, "Principles of Nourishment," *En-trophy Institute for Advanced Study* 1 (September–October 1978): 1–13.

3. Ross Hume Hall, "Thirty Years of Lassez-Faire in Human Nourishment," *En-trophy Institute for Advanced Study* 1 (March–April 1978): 9.

4. Ancel Keys, "Blood Lipids in Man: A Brief Review," *Journal of the American Dietetic Association* 51 (1967): 510.

5. Ross Hume Hall, "Cholesterol and Heart," *En-trophy Institute Review* 2 (September–October 1979): 14.

6. U. S. Department of Agriculture, Agricultural Research Service, *Nutrition Value of American Foods in Common Units*, by Catherine F. Adams, Agricultural Handbook No. 456 (Washington D.C.: Government Printing Office, 1975), pp. 231, 224.

7. Theodore P. Labuza, *Food and Your Well-Being* (New York: West Publishing Co., 1977), p. 72.

8. Ary J. Lamme III and Linda Leonard Lamme, "Children's Food Preferences," *The Journal of School Health* 50 (September 1980): 397.

9. Bruce R. Bistrian et al., "Advice on Nutrition," *New England Journal of Medicine* 304 (April 30, 1981): 1102.

Chapter 2

1. Nathaniel Hawthorne, *The House of the Seven Gables*, in *Familiar Quotations*, centennial ed., ed. John Bartlett (Boston: Little, Brown, 1955), p. 514a.

2. John Reis, psychotherapist, personal letter, December 1981. Personal Files of Betty Kamen, Cold Spring Harbor, New York.

3. Interview with Serafina Corsello, M.D., WMCA Radio, New York, November 1981.

4. Helen H. Gifft, Marjorie B. Washbon, and Gail G. Harrison, *Nutrition, Behavior and Change* (Englewood Cliffs, NJ: Prentice-Hall, 1972), p. 30.

5. Ibid., pp. 30, 36.

6. Michael Kamen, Education Consultant, personal letter, January 1982. Personal Files of Betty Kamen, Cold Spring Harbor, New York.

7. Robert B. Schafer, "Factors Affecting Food Behavior and the Quality of Husbands' and Wives' Diets," *Journal of the American Dietetic Association* 72 (February 1978): 138.

8. Ibid., p. 141.

9. Ary J. Lamme III and Linda Leonard Lamme, op. cit., p. 400.

10. Robert B. Schafer, op. cit., p. 115.

11. Helen H. Gifft, Marjorie B. Washbon, and Gail G. Harrison, op. cit., p. 38.

12. Select Committee on Nutrition and Human Needs, U.S. Senate, *Edible TV: Your Child and Food Commercials* (Washington, D.C.: Government Printing Office, September 1977), p. 69.

13. Ary J. Lamme III and Linda Leonard Lamme, op. cit., pp. 397–402.

14. Miriam E. Lowenberg et al., *Food and Man,* 2nd ed. (New York: John Wiley & Sons, 1974), p. 118.

15. Select Committee on Nutrition and Human Needs, U.S. Senate, op. cit., pp. 71–72.

16. Ross Hume Hall, "How Can We Feed the Hungry World? *En-trophy Institute Review* 2 (July–August 1979): 11

17. George McGovern, Foreword to Select Committee on Nutrition and Human Needs, U.S. Senate, op. cit., p. v.

18. Interview with Dr. Eva Snead, specializing in Nutrition and Holistic Medicine, WMCA Radio, New York, September 12, 1981.

19. John D. Kirschmann, *Nutrition Almanac* (New York: McGraw-Hill, 1973), p. 172.

20. E. M. E. Poskitt, T. J. Cole, and D. E. M. Lawson, "Diet, Sunlight and 25-hydroxy Vitamin D in Healthy Children and Adults," *British Medical Journal* 1 (January 1979): 223.

21. Marian Thompson Arlin, *The Science of Nutrition* (New York: Macmillan, 1972), p. 222.

22. Rudolph Ballentine, M.D., *Diet and Nutrition: A Holistic Approach* (Honesdale, PA: The Himalayan International Institute, 1978), p. 102.

23. Carl C. Pfeiffer, *Dr. Pfeiffer's Total Nutrition* (New York: Simon and Schuster, 1980), p. 62.

24. Theodore P. Labuza, *Food and Your Well-Being* (New York: West Publishing, 1977), p. 85.

25. George McGovern, Foreword to U.S. Senate Select Committee on Nutrition and Human Needs, op. cit., p. vi.

26. Ary J. Lamme III and Linda Leonard Lamme, op. cit., p. 400.

27. Select Committee on Nutrition and Human Needs, U.S. Senate, op. cit., p. 32.

28. Rudolph Ballentine, op. cit., p. 78.

29. John Yudkin, *Sweet and Dangerous* (New York: Peter H. Wyden, Inc., 1972), pp. 16–18.

30. Robert B. Schafer and Pat M. Keith, "Influences on Food Decisions Across the Family Life Cycle," *Journal of the American Dietetic Association* 78 (February 1981); 146.

31. Interview with Serafina Corsello, M.D., WMCA Radio, New York, November 1981.

32. Interview with Dr. Eva Snead, WMCA Radio, New York, September 12, 1981.

33. Robert B. Schafer, op. cit., pp. 141–42.

34. Helen H. Gifft, Marjorie B. Washbon, and Gail G. Harrison, op. cit., p. 254.

35. Interview with Serafina Corsello, M.D., WMCA Radio, New York, November 1981.

36. Select Committee on Nutrition and Human Needs, U.S. Senate, op. cit., p. 12.

37. Bonnie Britt, " 'Conscience' Battles Television Cavities," *Houston Chronicle,* September 18, 1981.

38. Ibid.

39. Ibid.

40. Documentary: *It's As Easy As Selling Candy to a Baby,* Action for Children's Television, Boston.

41. Interview with Peggy Charren, Action for Children's Television, September 19, 1981.

42. Sally Dussere, "The Effects of TV Advertising on Children's Eating Habits," thesis presented to the Department of Health, University of Massachusetts, 1976.

43. Select Committee on Nutrition and Human Needs, U.S. Senate, op. cit., p. 67; Witness Robert B. Choate.

44. Ibid., p. 26. Cross-examiner: Brenda Fox; Witness: Charles K. Atkin.

45. Ibid., p. 23. Witness: Kenneth George O'Bryan, November 15, 1976.

46. Documentary: *It's As Easy As Selling Candy to a Baby*, op. cit.

47. John Reis, psychotherapist, personal letter, December 1981. Personal Files of Betty Kamen, Cold Spring Harbor, New York.

48. Select Committee on Nutrition and Human Needs, U.S. Senate, op. cit., p. 36. Witness: George M. Owen, October 12, 1976.

49. Robert B. Schafer, op. cit., p. 141.

50. Select Committee on Nutrition and Human Needs, U.S. Senate, op. cit., p. 70.

Chapter 3

1. Emanuel Cheraskin, W. M. Ringsdorf, and Arline Brecker, *Psychodietetics: Food as the Key to Emotional Health* (New York: Stein and Day, 1974), p. 177.

2. J. Wayne MacFarland, "That Coffee Break Again," *Consumer Bulletin* (January 1968).

3. *A Complete Summary of the Iowa Breakfast Studies*, reported January 1976 by the Cereal Institute, 1111 Plaza Drive, Schaumburg, IL 60195.

4. Mark Mayell, "What Evils Lurk Behind All Those Vitamins?" *Nutrition Action* 8 (February 1981): 4–5.

5. John D. Kirschmann, *Nutrition Almanac* (New York: McGraw-Hill, 1973), p. 43.

6. Interview with Ross Hume Hall, Ph.D., Professor of Human Nutrition, McMaster University, Canada, June 5, 1978.

7. Karen MacNeil, *The Book of Whole Foods: Nutrition and Cuisine* (New York: Vintage Books, 1981), pp. 285–86.

8. Zenas Block, *It's All on the Label* (Boston: Little, Brown, 1981), p. 215.

9. Beatrice Trum Hunter, *Consumer Beware* (New York: Simon and Schuster, 1971), p. 268.

10. Gene Marine and Judith Van Allen, *Food Pollution: The Violation of Our Ecology* (New York: Holt, Rinehart & Winston, 1972), pp. 9–10.

11. Marian Thompson Arlin, *The Science of Nutrition* (New York: Macmillan, 1972), p. 26.

12. Richard J. Wurtman and Judith J. Wurtman, *Nutrition and the Brain*, Vol. 3 (New York: Raven Press, 1979), p. 213.

13. Carl C. Pfeiffer et al., *Mental and Elemental Nutrients: A Physician's Guide to Nutrition and Health Care* (New Canaan, CT: Keats Publishing, 1975).

14. Interview with Dr. C. Tom Smith, American Council of Applied Clinical Nutrition, WMCA Radio, New York, November 1981.

15. Jane Kinderlehrer, lecture presented at "Health and Nutrition Resources," Woodmere, New York, September 1978.

16. Fred A. Kummerow, "Mother Earth Versus the Food Industry," *Health Survival Digest* (February 1977): 1–3.

17. Ross Hume Hall, "Thirty Years of Laissez-Faire in Human Nourishment," *En-Trophy for Advanced Study* 3 (March–April, 1978):6.

18. American Medical Association Release, October 12, 1962.

19. George V. Mann, "Diet-Heart: End of an Era," *The New England Journal of Medicine* 297 (September 1977): 644.

20. Edward R. Gruberg and Stephen A. Raymond, *Beyond Cholesterol* (New York: St. Martin's Press, 1981), p. 30.

21. Rudolph Ballentine, *Diet and Nutrition: A Holistic Approach* (Honesdale, PA: The Himalayan International Institute, 1978), pp. 102–03.

22. Allen B. Nicols et al., "Independence on Serum Lipid Levels and Dietary Habits," *Journal of the American Medical Association* 236 (October 1976): 1948–53.

23. J. Hautuast, D. C. Bronsqeest-Schoute, and G. M. Dallinga-Thie, "The Effect on Serum Cholesterol of Removal of Eggs from the Diet of Free-Living Habitually Egg-Eating People," *American Journal of Clinical Nutrition* (November 1979): 2193–97.

24. A. Kamio, F. A. Kummerow, and H. Imai, "Degeneration of

Aortic Smooth Muscle Cells in Swine Fed Excess Vitamin D₃," *Archives of Pathological Laboratory Medicine* 101 (1977): 378.

25. Fred A. Kummerow and Harlan E. Moore, "Saturated Fat and Cholesterol Dietary 'Risk Factors' or Essentials to Human Life?" *Food and Nutrition News* (September–October 1981): 1–2.

26. Barbara Cooney O'Brien and Raymond Reiser, "Human Plasma Lipid Responses to Red Meat, Poultry, Fish, and Eggs," *The American Journal of Clinical Nutrition* 33 (December 1980): 2573.

27. Jon A. Story and David Kritchevsky, "Lignin and Bile Acid Binding," *Lancet* 2 (August 1981): 427.

28. O. J. Pollak, "Serum Cholesterol Levels Resulting from Various Egg Diets: Experimental Studies with Clinical Implications," *Journal of the American Geriatric Society* 6 (August 1958): 614–20.

29. Jeffrey Bland, *Your Health Under Siege: Using Nutrition to Fight Back*, (Brattleboro, VT: The Stephen Greene Press, 1981), p. 70.

30. John D. Kirschmann, Dir., *Nutrition Almanac* (New York: McGraw-Hill, 1973), p. 190.

31. Jacqueline Verrett and Jean Carper, *Eating May Be Hazardous to Your Health* (New York: Simon and Schuster, 1974), pp. 136–79.

32. "Proposal to Outlaw Nitrites," *Newsday,* August 18, 1978.

33. Interview with Paul Newberne, food scientist at Massachusetts Institute of Technology, WMCA Radio, New York, February 8, 1981.

34. Laurence N. Kolonel, M.D., et al., "Association of Diet and Place of Birth with Stomach Cancer Incidence in Hawaii: Japanese and Caucasians," *American Journal of Clinical Nutrition* 34 (November 1981): 2478–85.

35. T. Jukes, "Current Concepts in Nutrition," *New England Journal of Medicine* 297 (1977): 427.

36. Interview with Paul Newberne, food scientist at Massachusetts Institute of Technology, WMCA Radio, New York, February 8, 1981.

37. Benjamin T. Burton, *Human Nutrition* (New York: McGraw Hill, 1976), pp. 317–19.

38. Betty Kamen and Si Kamen, *The Kamen Plan for Total Nutrition During Pregnancy* (E. Norwalk, CT: Appleton-Century-Crofts, 1981), p. 46.

39. Ibid.

40. D. Ross, S. Sharnick, and K. A. Oster, *Proceedings of the Society of Experimental Biology in Medicine* 163 (January 1980): 141.

41. D. J. Ross, M. Praszynski, and K. A. Oster, *Proceedings of the Society of Experimental Biology in Medicine* 144 (1973): 523.

42. K. A. Oster, *St. Vincent/Park City Hospitals Medical Bulletin*, March 1973.

43. Interview with Dr. Lendon Smith, renowned author and pediatrician, WMCA Radio, New York, January 2, 1982.

44. Paul K. Stitt, biochemist and food scientist, personal letter, January 1982. Personal files of Betty Kamen, Cold Spring Harbor, New York.

45. Ross Hume Hall, *Food for Nought* (New York: Random House, 1976), pp. 9–34.

46. Beatrice Trum Hunter, *Consumer Beware*, op. cit., pp. 286–301.

47. Interview with Jane Kinderlehrer, Senior Editor of *Prevention Magazine*, Emmaus, PA, February 4, 1978.

48. Beatrice Trum Hunter, *The Great Nutrition Robbery* (New York: Charles Scribner's Sons, 1978), p. 132.

49. William Dufty, *Sugar Blues* (Radnor, PA: Chilton Book Company, 1975), p. 116.

50. Beatrice Trum Hunter, *The Great Nutrition Robbery*, op. cit., pp. 93–95.

51. Woodrow C. Monte, "Fiber: Its Nutritional Impact," *Journal of Applied Nutrition* 33 (1981): 71.

52. Code of Federal Regulations 21, *Food and Drugs*, Parts 100 to 199 (Washington, D.C.: U.S. Government Printing Office, 1977), p. 176.

53. Ruth Adams and Frank Murray, *The Good Seeds, The Rich Grains, The Hardy Nuts for a Healthier Happier Life* (New York: Larchmont Books, 1973), p. 196.

54. Ross Hume Hall, op. cit., pp. 9–34.

55. Richard A. Passwater, *Minerals and Your Health* (New Canaan, CT: Keats Publishing, Inc., 1980), p. 45, 192–93.

56. Paul A. Stitt with Mark Knickelbine and Scott Knickelbine, *Fighting the Food Giants* (Manitowec, WI: Natural Press, 1980), p. 83.

57. Donald R. Davis, "Wheat and Nutrition," *Nutrition Today* 16 (September–October 1981): 22–25.

58. John Reinhold, J. Salvador Garcia, and Pedro Garzoa, "Bind-

ing of Iron by Fiber of Wheat and Maize," *American Journal of Clinical Nutrition* 34 (July 1981): 1384–91.

59. Beatrice Trum Hunter, *Consumer Beware*, op. cit., p. 302.

60. Rudolph Ballentine, op. cit., p. 65.

61. Marlene Anne Bumgarner, *Book of Whole Grains* (New York: St. Martin's Press, 1976), pp. 53–54.

62. Magnus Pyke, *Technological Eating, or Where Does the Fish Finger Point?* (London: John Murray, 1972).

63. Ross Hume Hall, "The New Food Technology," *En-Trophy for Advanced Study* 3 (March–April, 1978):4.

64. Beatrice Trum Hunter, *The Great Nutrition Robbery*, op. cit., pp. 63–70.

65. Lecture by Beatrice Trum Hunter, Goddard Colloquium, Madison, CT, June 4, 1978.

66. Roslyn B. Alfin-Slater and Rose Mirenda, "Nutrient Requirements: What They Are and Bases for Recommendations," in *Human Nutrition: A Comprehensive Treatise*, Vol. 3A: *Nutrition and the Adult: Macronutrients*, gen. eds., Roslyn B. Alfin-Slater and David Kritchevsky (New York: Plenum Press, 1980), pp. 27–28.

67. "Girls' Pre-Teen Diet Tied to Breast Cancer," *Newsday*, September 9, 1976, p. 3.

68. Ross Hume Hall, *Food For Nought*, op. cit., p. 62.

69. Beatrice Trum Hunter, *Food Additives and Federal Policy: The Mirage of Safety* (New York: Charles Scribner's Sons, 1975), pp. 20–24.

70. Interview with Michael Jacobson, director of Center for Science in The Public Interest, WMCA Radio, New York, April 10, 1981.

71. Nutritional Scoreboard Poster, Center for Science in the Public Interest, Washington, D.C.

72. Beatrice Trum Hunter, *The Great Nutrition Robbery*, op. cit., p. 15.

73. Beatrice Trum Hunter, *Consumer Beware*, op. cit., pp. 201–208.

74. John Yudkin, *Sweet and Dangerous* (New York: Peter H. Wyden, Inc., 1972), p. 28.

75. T. L. Cleave, *The Saccharine Disease* (New Canaan, CT: Keats Publishing, Inc., 1974), pp. 180–86.

76. Ross Hume Hall, "Building Healthy Children Starting in the Womb," *En-Trophy Institute Review* 3 (January 1981): 14.

77. William Dufty, *Sugar Blues,* op. cit., p. 169.

78. Beatrice Trum Hunter, *Consumer Beware,* op. cit., pp. 244–45.

79. Code of Federal Regulations 21, *Food and Drugs,* Parts 100 to 199 (Washington, D.C.: U.S. Government Printing Office, 1977), p. 176.

80. Betty Kamen and Si Kamen, "The Protein Picture," from filmstrip series 922, *Exploding Nutrition Myths* (Garden City, NY: Bergwall Productions, 1979).

81. Marlene Anne Bumgarner, op. cit., p. 307.

82. Frances Moore Lappé, *Diet for a Small Planet* (New York: Ballantine Books, 1971), p. 157.

83. Catherine Fell, "Avocado: The Butter That Grows on Trees," *Bestways* (February 1977): 29–32.

84. Karen Cross Whyte, *The Complete Sprouting Cookbook* (San Francisco: Troubador Press, 1973), pp. 10–12, 28.

85. Helen H. Gifft, Marjorie B. Washbon, and Gail G. Harrison, *Nutrition, Behavior and Change* (Englewood Cliffs, NJ: Prentice-Hall, Inc., 1972), p. 265.

86. Ross Hume Hall, *Food for Nought,* op. cit., p. 49.

87. Carl C. Pfeiffer et al., *Mental and Elemental Nutrients: A Physician's Guide to Nutrition and Health Care* (New Canaan, CT: Keats Publishing, Inc., 1975), p. 5.

88. Ross Hume Hall, "Innovation Without Assessment," *En-Trophy for Advanced Study 3: Thirty Years of Laissez-Faire in Human Nutrition* (March–April 1978): 2, 5.

89. Jacqueline Verrett and Jean Carper, op. cit., p. 72.

90. Beatrice Trum Hunter, *Food Additives and Federal Policy: The Mirage of Safety,* op. cit., p. 14.

91. Interview with George Congram, Medical Nutritionist, Dix Hills, New York, August 1978.

92. Marlene Anne Bumgarner, op. cit., p. 185.

93. Ruth Adams and Frank Murray, op. cit., p. 81.

94. Marian Thompson Arlin, *The Science of Nutrition* (New York: Macmillan, 1972), p. 118.

95. Jim Mason and Peter Singer, *Animal Factories,* (New York: Crown Publishers, Inc., 1980), pp. 1–109.

96. Joan Gussow, lecture at Jo Giese Brown symposium, New York, June 23, 1981.

97. J. I. Rodale and staff, *Complete Book of Food And Nutrition* (Emmaus, PA: Rodale Press, 1972), p. 517.

98. Joseph M. Kadans, *"Encyclopedia of Fruits, Vegetables, Nuts and Seeds for Healthful Living* (West Nyack, NY: Parker Publishing, 1973), p. 123.

99. Ibid., p. 66.

100. Lecture and Nutrition Workshops, Hicksville, New York, February, 1976.

101. Carl C. Pfeiffer et al., op. cit., pp. 385–90.

102. "Gourmet Foods Now TV Dinners," *Wall Street Journal,* May 5, 1967.

103. Lecture by Ross Hume Hall, Goddard College Colloquium, Madison, CT, April 6, 1978.

104. Philip Chen, *Mineral Balance In Eating For Health* (Emmaus, PA: Rodale Press, 1969), p. xiii.

105. Richard Passwater, *Supernutrition for Healthy Hearts* (New York: Dial Press, 1977), p. 144.

106. "Can't Seem to Shake It," *Well-Being* 35 (August 15, 1978):6.

107. Benjamin H. Ershoff, "Effects of the Dietary Sodium: Potassium Ratio in the Treatment of Hypertension," *Journal of Applied Nutrition* 33 (1981): 161.

108. "Salt and Hypertension," *Nutrition Action* 8 (April 1981): 3–4.

109. Beatrice Trum Hunter, *Consumer Beware*, op. cit., p. 198.

110. *Nutrition Action* 7 (December 1980): 5.

111. J. I. Rodale and staff, *Complete Book of Food and Nutrition,* op. cit., pp. 352–59.

112. Joanne Moyer, *Nuts and Seeds: the Natural Snacks* (Emmaus, PA: Rodale Press, 1973), pp. 29–36.

113. Jacqueline Verrett and Jean Carper, op. cit., p. 221.

114. Frank L. Iber, "In Alcohol, the Liver Sets the Pace," *Nutrition Today* (January–February 1971): 2–9.

115. J. I. Rodale and staff, *Best Health Articles* (Emmaus, PA: Rodale Press, 1967), pp. 285, 858.

116. Personal correspondence with the Norwegian Dairies Sales Association, Oslo, Norway, March 31, 1977.

117. Gene Marine and Judith Van Allen, op. cit., pp. 47–48.

118. Beatrice Trum Hunter, *Consumer Beware*, op. cit., pp. 247–49.

119. Ross Hume Hall, "Building Healthy Children Starting in the Womb," *En-Trophy Institute Review* 3 (January 1981): 15.

Chapter 4

1. Myron Winick, ed., *Current Concepts in Nutrition,* Vol. 2: *Nutrition and Fetal Development* (New York: John Wiley & Sons, 1974), p. 20.

2. Ross Hume Hall, "Building Healthy Children Starting in the Womb," *En-trophy Institute Review* 3 (1980): 3.

3. Ross Hume Hall, "Building Healthy Children Starting in the Womb," op. cit., p. 7.

4. H. Marano, "Breast Feeding: New Evidence: It's Far More Than Nutrition," *Medical World News,* February 5, 1979, pp. 62–78.

5. S. J. Fomon and R. G. Strauss, *New England Journal of Medicine* 299 (1978): 355–57.

6. D. B. Jelliffe and E. F. P. Jelliffe, "The Uniqueness of Human Milk," *American Journal of Clinical Nutrition* 24 (1971): 968–69.

7. S. R. Halpern et al., "Development of Childhood Allergy in Infants Fed Breast, Soy or Cow Milk," *Clinical Immunology* 51 (March 1973): 139–51.

8. J. Michael Gurney, "The Problems of Feeding the Weaning Age Group: An Overview of Available Solutions," *Cajanus* 12 (1979): 43.

9. Calvin W. Woodruff, "Supplementary Food for Infants," *Contemporary Nutrition* 6 (January 1981): 1.

10. Betty Kamen and Si Kamen, *The Kamen Plan for Total Nutrition During Pregnancy* (E. Norwalk, CT: Appleton-Century-Crofts, 1981), pp. 31–50.

11. Jose Villar and Jose M. Belizan, "Breastfeeding in Developing Countries," *Lancet* 2 (September 1981): 622.

12. Emory W. Thurston, *Nutrition for Tots to Teens* (Calabasas, CA: Institute of Nutritional Research, 1976), p. 33.

13. Alvin N. Eden, *Positive Parenting* (New York: Bobbs-Merrill, 1980), p. 125.

14. Lendon Smith, *Feed Your Kids Right* (New York: McGraw-Hill, 1979), p. 223.

15. Derrick B. Jelliffe and E. F. Patrice Jelliffe, *Human Milk in the Modern World* (New York: Oxford University Press, 1978), p. 406.

16. C. T. Smith, director of the American Council of Applied Clinical Nutrition, WMCA Radio interview, January 30, 1982.

17. Archie Kalokerinos, *Every Second Child* (New Canaan, CT: Keats Publishing, Inc., 1981), pp. 97–98.

18. Calvin W. Woodruff, "Supplementary Food for Infants," *Contemporary Nutrition* 6 (January 1981): 1.

19. Guy H. Johnson, George A. Purvis, and Robert D. Wallace, "What Nutrients Do Our Infants Really Get?" *Nutrition Today* 16 (July–August): 5.

20. S. Bachrach, J. Fisher, and J. S. Parks, "An Outbreak of Vitamin D Deficiency Rickets in a Susceptible Population," *Pediatrics* 64 (1979): 871–77.

21. Committee on Nutrition, American Academy of Pediatrics, "Commentary on Breast-Feeding and Infant Formulas, Including Proposed Standards for Formulas," *Pediatrics* 57 (1976): 278–85.

22. Guy H. Johnson, George A. Purvis, and Robert D. Wallace, "What Nutrients Do Our Infants Really Get?" *Nutrition Today* 16 (July–August 1981): 5.

23. Derrick B. Jelliffe and E. F. Patrice Jelliffe, op. cit., p. 80.

24. Robert L. Jackson, "Maternal and Infant Nutrition and Health in Later Life," *Nutrition Reviews*, 37 (February 1979):35.

25. J. Michael Gurney, "The Problems of Feeding the Weaning Age Group: An Overview of Available Solutions," *Cajanus* 12 (1979): 43–51.

26. Beatrice Trum Hunter, personal letter of October 19, 1981. Personal Files of Betty Kamen, Cold Spring Harbor, New York.

27. Ross Hume Hall, "Building Healthy Children Starting in the Womb," op. cit., p. 11.

28. Tom Monte, "Warning: Honey May Be Hazardous to Your Infant, *Nutrition Action* (September 1979): 10.

29. "School Lunch: Time to Act," *Nutrition Action* (September 1976): 4.

30. Sara Sloan, director of food service, Atlanta, Georgia, in personal letter, May 1979. Personal files of Betty Kamen, Cold Spring Harbor, New York.

31. Interview with Lendon Smith, M.D., WMCA Radio, New York, October 17, 1981.

32. Letter from Jerome Vogel, Nutrition Director, New York Institute of Technology, to Betty Kamen, January 1982. Personal files of Betty Kamen, Cold Spring Harbor, New York.

33. John I. McKigney and Hamish N. Munro, eds., *Nutrient Requirements in Adolescence* (Cambridge, MA: MIT Press, 1976), p. 132.

34. Barry Lauton and Arthur S. Freese, *The Healthy Adolescent* (New York: Charles Scribner's Sons, 1981), p. 144.

35. C. Trevor Greenwood and David P. Richardson, "Nutrition During Adolescence," *World Review of Nutrition and Dietetics* 33 (1979): 22.

36. Charlotte Christensen Cook and Irene R. Payne, "Effect of Supplements on the Nutrient Intake of Children," *Journal of the American Dietetic Association* 74 (1979): 132–33.

37. C. Trevor Greenwood and David P. Richardson, op. cit., pp. 33–34.

38. Ander Hager, "Nutritional Problems in Adolescence-Obesity," *Nutrition Reviews* 39 (February 1981): 89–95.

39. William Shakespeare, *As You Like It.*

40. Robert C. Atkins, *Dr. Atkins' Nutritional Breakthrough* (New York: William Morrow and Company, 1981), p. 144.

41. Denis Burkitt, *Eat Right to Stay Healthy and Enjoy Life More* (New York: Arco Publishing, Inc., 1979), p. 101.

42. Jonathan V. Wright, *Dr. Wright's Book of Nutritional Therapy* (Emmaus, PA: Rodale Press, 1979), p. 6.

43. U.S. Select Committee on Nutrition and Human Needs, *Dietary Goals for the United States,* 2nd ed., (Washington, D.C.: Government Printing Office, December 1977), p. 20.

44. Ibid. (February 1977), p. 9.

45. H. L. Newbold, *Mega-Nutrients for Your Nerves* (New York: Peter H. Wyden, 1975), p. 17.

46. Edward James Calabrese, *Nutrition and Environmental Health,* Vol. 1: *The Vitamins* (New York: John Wiley and Sons, 1980), pp. 250–51.

47. U.S. Select Committee on Nutrition and Human Needs (December 1977), op. cit., p. 38.

48. D. M. Hegsted, "Optimal Nutrition," *Cancer* 43 (May 1979): 1996.

49. Jeffrey Bland, "Endocrinology and Adolescent Nutrition," *Journal of Applied Nutrition* 33 (1981): 156–59.

50. Charlotte Christensen Cook and Irene R. Payne, op. cit., pp. 130–33.

51. N. I. Max Kjellman, "Effect of Parental Smoking on IgE Levels in Children," *Lancet* 1 (2 May 1981): 993–94.

52. Betty Kamen and Si Kamen, op. cit., p. 47.

53. Edward James Calabrese, op. cit., p. 71.

54. Benjamin T. Burton, *Human Nutrition* (New York: McGraw-Hill, 1976), pp. 490–513.

55. Myron Winick, *Nutrition In Health and Disease*, op. cit., pp. 107–08.

56. Earl Mindell, *Earl Mindell's Vitamin Bible for Your Kids* (New York: Rawson, Wade, 1981), p. 116.

57. Ananda S. Prasad, "Nutritional Zinc Today," *Nutrition Today* 16 (March–April 1981): 4–12.

58. K. Michael Hambidge et al., "Zinc Nutritional Status of Young Middle-Income Children and Effects of Consuming Zinc-Fortified Breakfast Cereals," *American Journal of Clinical Nutrition* 32 (December 1979): 2532.

59. Emil Ginter, "Chronic Marginal Vitamin C Deficiency: Biochemistry and Pathophysiology," *World Review of Nutrition and Dietetics* 33 (1979): 105.

60. Richard A. Kunin, *Mega Nutrition* (New York: McGraw-Hill, 1980), p. 98.

61. Earl Mindell, *Earl Mindell's Vitamin Bible for Your Kids* (New York: Rawson, Wade Publishers, 1981), p. 116.

62. James C. S. Kim, "Nutrient-Pollutant Interaction: Animals as Monitors of Nutritional Deficiencies," *Journal of Applied Nutrition* 33 (1981): 114.

63. Malathi Damodaran et al., "Vitamin B-complex Deficiency and Visual Acuity," *British Journal of Nutrition* 41 (1979): 41.

64. A. I. Mendeloff, "Current Concepts: Dietary Fiber and Human Health," *New England Journal of Medicine* 297 (1977): 811.

65. Denis Burkitt, op. cit., p. 101.

66. American Academy of Pediatrics: Committee on Nutrition, "Plant Fiber Intake in the Pediatric Diet," *Pediatrics* 67 (April 1981): 573.

67. Patricia A. Judd and A. Stewart Truswell, "The Effect of

Rolled Oats in Blood Lipids and Fecal Steroid Excretion in Man,"
American Journal of Clinical Nutrition 34 (October 1981): 1061–67.

68. Sheldon E. Schwartz and Gary D. Levine, "Effects of Dietary
Fiber on Intestinal Glucose Absorption and Glucose Tolerance in
Rats," *Gastroenterology* 79 (November 1980): 836.

69. G. B. Haber, K. W. Heaton, and D. Murphy, "Depletion and
Disruption of Dietary Fiber," *Lancet* (1 October 1977): 679–82.

70. Kerin O'Dea, Penelope Snow, and Paul Nestel, "Rate of
Starch Hydrolysis in Vitro as a Predictor of Metabolic Responses to
Complete Carbohydrate in Vivo," *American Journal of Clinical Nutrition* 34 (October 1981): 1991–93.

71. Irma H. Ullrich et al., "Alterations of Fecal Steroid Composition Induced by Changes in Dietary Fiber Consumption," *American Journal of Clinical Nutrition* 34 (October 1981): 2054–59.

72. Donald R. Davis, "Wheat and Nutrition, Part I," *Nutrition Today* 16 (July–August 1981): 16–21.

73. C. Bhaskaram and Vinodini Reddy, "Role of Dietary Phytate
in the Aetiology of Nutritional Rickets," *Indian Journal of Medical Research* 69 (1979): 265.

74. Eugene R. Morris and Rex Ellis, "Isolation of Monoferric
Phytate from Wheat Bran and Its Biological Value as an Iron Source
to the Rat," *Journal of Nutrition* 106 (1976): 753–59.

75. Ibid., p. 759.

76. D. G. H. Daniels and N. Fisher, "Hydrolysis of the Phytate of
Wheat Flour During Breadmaking," *British Journal of Nutrition* 46
(July 1981): 1–6.

77. Howard Jacobson, *Racewalk to Fitness* (New York: Simon
and Schuster, 1980), p. 223.

78. Helen H. Gifft, Marjorie B. Washbon, and Gail G. Harrison,
Nutrition, Behavior and Change (Englewood Cliffs, NJ: Prentice-Hall,
1972), p. 281.

79. E. M. E. Poskitt, T. J. Cole, and D. E. M. Lawson, "Diet,
Sunlight and 25-Hydroxy Vitamin D in Healthy Children and Adults,"
British Medical Journal 1 (January 1979): 221–23.

80. Russell W. Chesney et al., "Serum I, 25 Dihydroxyvitamin D
Levels in Normal Children and In Vitamin D Disorders," *American Journal of Disabled Children* 134 (February 1980): 135–39.

81. "The Active Form of Vitamin D Stimulates the Synthesis of a

Vitamin K-Dependent Bone Protein," *Nutrition Reviews* 39 (July 1981): 135–39.

82. William C. MacLean and George G. Graham, "Vegetarianism in Children," *American Journal of Disabled Children* 134 (May 1980): 513–19.

83. Johanna T. Dwyer et al., "Mental Age and I.Q. of Predominately Vegetarian Children," *Journal of the American Dietetic Association* 76 (1980): 142–47.

84. Vilma T. Falck, "Application of the Behavioral Sciences to Dietary Practices," *Nutrition Today* 16 (May–June 1981): 29.

Chapter 5

1. William G. Crook, "Can What a Child Eats Make Him Dull, Stupid, or Hyperactive?" *Journal of Learning Disabilities* 13 (May 1980): 285.

2. N.Y. Institute for Child Development, Inc., *Reaching Children Bulletin* (New York, NY: 1981), pp. 2–3.

3. Charlotte Hutchens, "Subtracting Additives," *Journal of Practical Nursing* 29 (July 1979): 13–14.

4. Bernard Rimland and Gerald E. Larson, "Nutritional and Ecological Approaches to the Reduction of Criminality, Delinquency and Violence," *Journal of Applied Nutrition* 33 (1981): 118.

5. Arnold J. Sameroff, "Early Influences on Development: Fact or Fancy?" *Merrill-Palmer Quarterly* 21 (1975): 269.

6. Bonnie F. Liebman and Greg Moyer, "The Case Against Sugar," *Nutrition Action* 7 (December 1980): 12.

7. William G. Crook, op. cit., p. 283.

8. Ibid.

9. N.Y. Institute for Child Development, Inc., *Reaching Children Bulletin,* (New York, NY: n. d.,), p. 2

10. J. M. Swanson and M. Kinsbourne, "Food Dyes Impair Performance of Hyperactive Children on a Laboratory Learning Test," *Science* 207 (1980): 1485–87.

11. William G. Crook, op. cit., pp. 284–85.

12. Arnold Brenner, "Trace Mineral Levels in Hyperactive Chil-

dren Responding to the Feingold Diet," *Journal of Pediatrics* 94 (June 1979): 944–45.

13. Interview with Lendon Smith, M.D., WMCA Radio, New York, January 2, 1982.

14. Ninfa Saturnino Springer, "Ascorbic Acid Status of Children with Development Disabilities," *Journal of the American Dietetic Association* 75 (October 1979): 425–28.

15. G. A. Glugston, "The Effect of Malnutrition on Brain Growth and Intellectual Development," *The Tropical Doctor* 2 (January 1981): 32–38.

16. Bernard Rimland and Gerald E. Larson, "Nutrition and Ecological Approaches to the Reduction of Criminality, Delinquency, and Violence," *Journal of Applied Nutrition*, 33 (1981):127.

17. R. F. Harrel et al., "Can Nutritional Supplements Help Mentally Retarded Children? An Exploratory Study," *Proceedings of the National Academy of Sciences* 78 (January 1981): 574–78.

18. Bernard Rimland and Gerald E. Larson, op. cit., p. 132.

19. H. Hafer, *Nahrungsphosphat als Ursache fur Uerhaltensstorugen und Jugend Kriminalitat* (Heidlberg, Kriminalistik Verlag, 1979).

20. Interview with Lendon Smith, M.D., WMCA Radio, New York, January 2, 1982.

21. Benjamin T. Burton, *Human Nutrition,* 3rd ed. (New York: McGraw-Hill, 1976), pp. 490–513.

22. William G. Crook, op. cit., 281.

23. Helen Tryphonas and Ronald Trites, "Blood Levels of Antibodies to Specific Foods," *Annals of Allergy* 42 (1979): 22.

24. D. S. King, "Can Allergic Exposure Provoke Psychological Symptoms? A Double-Blind Test," *Biological Psychiatry* 16 (1981): 3–19.

25. Alexander Schauss, *Diet, Crime and Delinquency* (Berkeley, CA: Parker House, 1980), pp. 80–81.

26. Ibid., p. 85.

27. Arnold Brenner, "Trace Mineral Levels in Hyperactive Children Responding to the Feingold Diet," *Journal of Pediatrics* 94 (June 1979): 944–45.

28. Ifor D. Capel et al., "Comparison of Concentrations of Some Trace, Bulk, and Toxic Metals in the Hair of Normal and Dyslexic Children," *Clinical Chemistry* 27 (1981): 879–81.

29. O. J. David et al., "Lead and Hyperactivity: Behavioral Response to Chelation: A Pilot Study," *American Journal of Psychiatry* 133 (October 1976): 1155–58.

30. Mark Mayell, "Why There Is Lead in Your Soup," *Environment and Behavior* 1 (February 1981): 6.

31. R. O. Pihl and M. Parkes, "Hair Element Content in Learning Disabled Children," *Science* 198 (1977): 204–06.

32. Herbert L. Needleman et al., "Deficits in Psychologic and Classroom Performance of Children with Elevated Dentine Lead Levels," *New England Journal of Medicine* 300 (March 29, 1979): 689–95.

33. Alexander Schauss, op. cit., p. 35.

34. Carl C. Pfeiffer, *Mental and Elemental Nutrients: A Physician's Guide to Nutrition and Health Care* (New Canaan, CT: Keats Publishing, Inc., 1975), pp. 131–32.

35. John D. Kirschmann, *Nutrition Almanac* (New York: McGraw-Hill, 1975), p. 72.

36. Denis Burkitt, *Eat Right to Stay Healthy and Enjoy Life More* (New York: Arco Publishing, Inc., 1979), p. 43.

37. J. B. Shields and H. H. Mitchell, "The Effect of Calcium and Phosphorous on the Metabolism of Lead," *Journal of Nutrition* 21 (1941): 541.

38. Edward James Calabrese, *Nutrition and Environmental Health*, vol. 2, *Minerals and Macronutrients* (New York: John Wiley and Sons, 1981), pp. 192, 356–57.

39. Ibid., pp. 59–60.

40. R. W. Chadwick, M. F. Copeland, and C. J. Chadwick, "Enhanced Pesticide Metabolism: A Previously Unreported Effect of Dietary Fibre in Mammals," *Food, Cosmetics and Toxicology* 16 (1978): 217–25.

41. Edward James Calabrese, op cit., p. 393.

42. Ibid., p. 61.

43. American Academy of Pediatrics, *Proceedings of Conference on Susceptibility Chemical Pollutants* (Browns Lake, WI: 1973), p. 857.

44. Ibid., p. 858.

45. John N. Ott, "Responses of Psychological and Physiological Functions to Environmental Light: Part 1," *Journal of Learning Disabilities* 1 (June 1968): pp. 6–12, 18–20.

46. Gina Bari Koleta, "Behavioral Teratology: Birth Defects of the Mind," *Science* 202 (1978): 732–34.

47. Joe Graedon with Teresa Graedon, *The People's Pharmacy: 2* (New York: Avon Books, 1980), p. 315.

48. Richard M. Carlton, "Some Foods and Environmental Substances That Affect Behavior." New York (mimeographed).

49. Alan K. Done, Summer J. Yaffe, and John M. Clayton, "Aspirin Dosage for Infants," *Journal of Pediatrics* 95 (1979): 617–24.

Chapter 6

1. Michael A. Weiner, *Earth Medicine: Earth Foods* (New York: Macmillan, 1972), p. 72.

2. Paul M. Kourennoff and George St. George, *Russian Folk Medicine*, (New York: Pyramid Books, 1971), p. 153.

3. Lelord Kordel, *Natural Folk Remedies* (New York: G.P. Putnam's Sons, 1974), p. 78–79.

4. Aaron E. Ifekwunigwe et al., "Immune Response to Measles and Smallpox Vaccinations in Malnourished Children," *American Journal of Clinical Nutrition* 33 (March 1980): 621–24.

5. Vilma T. Falck, "Application of the Behavioral Sciences to Dietary Practices," *Nutrition Today* 16 (May–June 1981): 28.

6. Lucretius, "De Rerum Natura," IV: 637, in *Familiar Quotations,* centennial ed., ed. John Bartlett (Boston: Little, Brown, 1955), p. 34b.

7. P. D. Buisseret, "Common Manifestations of Cow's Milk Allergy in Children," *Lancet* 1 (February 11, 1978): 304–05.

8. Irene Jakobsson and Tor Linberg, "Cow's Milk as a Cause of Infantile Colic in Breast-fed Infants," *Lancet* 2 (August 26, 1978): 437–39.

9. William Kaufman, "Food-Induced Allergic Illness in Children," *International Archives of Allergy and Applied Immunology* 13 (1958): 68–101.

10. "Allergy/Immunology," *Postgraduate Medicine* 67 (March 1980): 71.

11. William C. Deamer, John W. Gerrard, and Frederic Speer,

"Cow's Milk Allergy: A Critical Review," *Journal of Family Practice* 9 (August 1979): 223–32.

12. Robert S. Goodhart and Maurice E. Shils, eds., *Modern Nutrition in Health and Disease*, 6th ed. (Philadelphia: Lea and Febiger, 1980), pp. 1080–81.

13. Emanuel Lebenthal, *Textbook of Gastroenterology and Nutrition in Infancy*, Vol. 2 (New York: Raven Press, 1981), p. 703.

14. Ibid., p. 705.

15. Lelord Kordel, op. cit., pp. 183–84.

16. Harold Ilecks, "Anaphylaxis from Milk Protein in Diaper Ointment," *Journal of the American Medical Association* 244 (October 3, 1980): 1560.

17. Don Mannerberg and June Roth, *Aerobic Nutrition* (New York: Hawthorn/Dutton, 1981), pp. 56–57.

18. William G. Crook, *Your Allergic Child* (Jackson, TN: Pedicenter Press, 1974), p. 140.

19. "Food Allergy," *Lancet* 1 (February 3, 1979): 249.

20. Don Mannerberg and June Roth, op. cit., pp. 56–57.

21. William G. Crook, op. cit., pp. 142–44.

22. Don Mannerberg and June Roth, op. cit., pp. 56–57.

23. William G. Crook, op. cit., p. 146.

24. Don Mannerberg and June Roth, op. cit., pp. 56–57.

25. William G. Crook, op. cit., pp. 141–42.

26. William R. Holub, "Do Allergic Reactions Represent Hypersensitivity or Nutritionally Deficient Detoxification?" *Journal of Applied Nutrition* 31 (1979): 67–74.

27. Lelord Kordel, op. cit., pp. 121, 141.

28. Jonathan V. Wright, *Dr. Wright's Book of Nutritional Therapy*, Emmaus, PA: Rodale Press, 1979), pp. 49–50.

29. Emory W. Thurston, *Nutrition for Tots to Teens* (Calabasas, CA: Institute of Nutritional Research, 1976), p. 134–36.

30. Tatsuo Matsumura et al., "Egg Sensitivity and Eczematous Manifestations in Breast-fed Newborns with Particular Reference to Intrauterine Sensitization," *Annals of Allergy* 35 (October 1975): 221–29.

31. Benjamin F. Miller and Clair Brickman Keane, *Encylopedia and Dictionary of Medicine, Nursing, and Allied Health*, 2nd ed. (Philadelphia: W. B. Saunders Company, 1978), p. 321.

32. P. C. Jackson et al., "Intestinal Permeability in Patients with Eczema and Food Allergy," *Lancet* 1 (June, 13 1981): 1285–86.

33. "Food Allergy," *Lancet* 1 (February 3, 1979): 249.

34. Jonathan V. Wright, op. cit., p. 45.

35. Lendon Smith, *Feed Your Kids Right* (New York: McGraw-Hill Book Company, 1979), p. 43.

36. Carl C. Pfeiffer, *Mental and Elemental Nutrients* (New Canaan, CT: Keats Publishing Inc., 1975), p. 235.

37. Jonathan V. Wright, op. cit., p. 35.

38. Lendon Smith, op. cit., p. 96.

39. Emanuel Cheraskin, "Sucrose, Neutrophilic Phagocytosis and Resistance to Disease," *Dental Surgery* 52 (December 1976): 46–48.

40. G. J. Ebrahim, "The Problems of Undernutrition," in *Nutrition and Disease*, ed. R. J. Jarrett (Baltimore: University Park Press, 1979), p. 31.

41. John R. K. Robson, *Malnutrition: It's Causation and Control* (New York: Gordon and Breach, 1972), p. 40.

42. O. P. Ghai and V. P. Choudhry, "Nutritional Anemia in Children," *Pediatrician* 9 (1980): 113–26.

43. G. J. Ebrahim, op. cit., pp. 118–29.

44. "An Evaluation of Children with Gluten-Sensitive Enteropathy: Clinical and Laboratory Data Compared with Jejunal Biopsy Findings," *Nutrition Reviews* 39 (October 1981): 365–68.

45. W. K. Dicke, H. A. Weijers, and J. H. Van de Kamer, "An Evaluation of Children with Gluten Sensitive Enteropathy: Clinical and Laboratory Data Compared with Jujunal Biopsy Findings," *Acta Pediatrics* 42 (1953): 34–42.

46. J. Gryboski, "False Security of A Gluten-Free Diet," *American Journal of Diseases of Children* 135 (February, 1981): 110–111.

47. Azaria Ashkenazi et al., "Effect of Gluten-Free Diet on an Immunological Assay for Celiac Disease," *Lancet* 1 (April 25, 1981): 914–16.

48. J. Kokkonen and S. Simila, "Gastric Function and Absorption of Vitamin B_{12} in Children with Celiac Disease," *European Journal of Pediatrics* 132 (October 1979): 71–75.

49. "Response of Gluten-Sensitive Enteropathy to Corticosteroids," *Nutrition Reviews* 39 (March 1981): 132–34.

50. J. J. Littlewood and Avril J. Crollick, "Childhood Celiac Dis

ease is Disappearing," *Lancet* 2 (December 1980): 1359.

51. Katherine M. Dormandy, A. H. Waters, and D. L. Mollin, "Folic Acid Deficiency in Celiac Disease," *Lancet* 1 (March 23, 1963): 632–35.

52. Benjamin T. Burton, *Human Nutrition* (New York: McGraw-Hill, 1976), p. 117.

53. Richard A. Kunin, *Mega-Nutrition* (New York: McGraw-Hill, 1980), p. 241.

54. John R. Christopher, *Childhood Diseases* (Springville, UT: Christopher Publications, 1978), pp. 49–50, 176.

55. Thomas A. Anderson, "Commercial Infant Foods: Content and Composition," *Pediatric Clinics of North America* 24 (February 1977): 40.

56. Carl C. Pfeiffer, op. cit., p. 125.

57. Rudolph Ballentine, *Diet and Nutrition: A Holistic Approach* (Honesdale, PA: The Himalayan International Institute, 1978), p. 199.

58. Geoffrey H. Bourne, "Vitamin C and Immunity," *British Journal of Nutrition* 2 (1949): 345.

59. Virginia W. Livingston, *Cancer: A New Breakthrough* (San Diego: Reward Books, 1979).

60. Robert C. Atkins, *Dr. Atkins' Nutritional Breakthrough* (New York: William Morrow and Company, 1981), pp. 145–47.

61. Rudolph Ballentine, op. cit., p. 199.

62. Carl C. Pfeiffer, *Zinc and Other Micro-Nutrients* (New Canaan, CT: Keats Publishing, Inc., 1978), p. 52.

63. John D. Kirschmann, *Nutrition Almanac* (New York: McGraw-Hill, 1973), pp. 32, 143.

64. James D'Adamo with Allan Richards, *One Man's Food* (New York: Richard Marek Publishers, 1980), p. 195.

65. Rudolph Ballentine, op. cit., p. 202.

66. Dian Dincin Buchman, *Herbal Medicine* (New York: David McKay, 1979), pp. 131–32.

67. Ibid., pp. 176–77.

68. Ibid., p. 46.

69. Ibid.

70. "Critical Issues In Human Nutrition Research and Research Training in the 1980s," *American Journal of Clinical Nutrition* 34 (May 1981): 1003–1004.

71. Select Committee on Nutrition and Human Needs; U.S. Senate, *Edible TV: Your Child and Food Commercials* (Washington, D.C.: Government Printing Office, September 1977), p. 40.

72. Denis Burkitt, *Eat Right to Stay Healthy* (New York: Arco Publishing, Inc., 1979), p. 49.

73. Rubin Bressler, Morton D. Bogdonoff, and Genell J. Subak-Sharpe, eds., *The Physician's Drug Manual: Prescription and Nonprescription Drugs* (Garden City, NY: Doubleday and Company, Inc., 1980), p. 264.

74. Ibid.

75. Emory W. Thurston, op. cit., p. 79.

76. Norbert Hirschhorn, "The Treatment of Acute Diarrhea in Children: An Historical and Physiological Perspective," *American Journal of Clinical Nutrition* 33 (March 1980): 637–63.

77. H. Marchovitch, "Leopamide in 'Toddler Diarrhea,' " *Lancet* 1 (June 28, 1980): 1413.

78. Fima Lifshitz and Marjorie Marks-Katz, "Treatment for Diarrhea," paper prepared especially for this book, January 1982.

79. John Christopher, *Childhood Diseases* (Springfield, UT: Christopher Publications, 1978), p. 64.

80. James D'Adamo with Allan Richards, op. cit., p. 202.

81. Robert C. Atkins, op. cit., p. 125.

82. James D'Adamo with Allan Richards, op. cit., p. 203.

83. Ellen Grant, "Food Allergy and Migraine," *Lancet* 1 (May 5, 1979): 966–68.

84. J. Monro et al., "Food Allergy in Migraine," *Lancet* 2 (1980): 1–4.

85. Dian Dincin Buchman, op. cit., p. 208.

86. Interview with David F. Horrobin, M.D., research scientist, WMCA Radio, New York, September 26, 1981.

87. Colm O'Herlihy, "Jogging and Suppression of Ovulation," *Lancet* 1 (January 7, 1982): 50–51.

Chapter 7

1. C. K. Lyon, "Sesame: Current Knowledge of Composition and Use," *Journal of Oil Chemical Society* 49 (1972): 245.

2. Alpasian Peheivanturk, Ankara, Turkey, via Turkish Embassy, Washington, D.C.

3. Jonathan V. Wright, *Dr. Wright's Book of Nutritional Therapy* (Emmaus, PA: Rodale Press, 1979), p. 30.

4. Judith J. Wurtman, *Eating Your Way Through Life* (New York: Raven Press, 1979), p. 22.

5. Thomas Henry Huxley, "Technical Education," in *Familiar Quotations,* centennial ed., ed. John Bartlett (Boston: Little, Brown, 1955), p. 634a.

6. Rudolph Ballentine, *Diet and Nutrition* (Honesdale, PA: The Himalayan International Institute, 1978), p. 53.

7. American Academy of Pediatrics, Committee on Nutrition, "Pediatrics: Plant Fiber Intake in the Pediatric Diet," *Pediatrics* 67 (April 1981): 572–75.

8. R. J. Jarrett, *Nutrition and Disease* (Baltimore: University Park Press, 1979), p. 24.

9. William Wordsworth, "The Tables Turned," Stanza 4, in *Familiar Quotations,* op. cit., p. 403b.

FOOD AND NUTRITION GLOSSARY

ACIDOPHILUS—A milk product containing viable bacteria which, when present in the intestine, increases efficiency.

AMINO ACIDS—The component parts of protein, often referred to as "the building blocks of protein."

ASSIMILATION—The change of digested food into the cells of an animal.

BIOFLAVONOIDS—A compound that helps maintain the capillary walls, reducing the likelihood of hemorrhaging.

ANEMIA—A condition caused by a reduced number of red blood cells. Anemia is not a disease, but a symptom of several different disorders. It may be caused by poor diet, loss of blood, industrial poisons, or any of several other conditions.

BIOAVAILABILITY—The degree to which a substance is available to the body.

CALORIE—A calorie is a unit used to express an amount of food able to produce one large calorie of energy. It is possible to calculate the amount of energy contained in a particular food by measuring the amount of heat units, or calories, in that food.

CERTIFIED RAW MILK—Milk that is not heated before being sold and is certified to be safe for human use.

CHOLESTEROLEMIA—High cholesterol levels in the blood.

DESICCATED LIVER—A food supplement made from liver from which the lining, connective tissue and fat has been removed. A rich source of iron and B-complex.

DETOXIFY—Removal of poisons from the body.

DIET—What a person eats and drinks.

ESSENTIAL FATTY ACIDS—A family of organic fats that cannot be produced in the body. They must be obtained from food.

FIBER—The indigestible parts of food.

FLUORIDE—A compound of the element fluorine; fluorides in small quantities are essential nutrients, strengthening the bones and teeth.

GLUCOSE—A simple sugar found in foodstuffs, especially fruit, and in normal blood; chief energy source for living organisms.

GRAIN—A small hard seedlike fruit of any cereal plant.

HOMOGENIZED—Processing of milk so that fat particles are finely divided and emulsified to prevent the cream from separating on standing.

HORMONE—A substance formed in some organ of the body and carried by the body fluid to another organ or tissue where it has a specific effect.

HYDROGENATION—Adding hydrogen to fat molecules (oil is hydrogenated to produce a solid fat).

HYPERTENSION—Persistently high blood pressure.

LACTASE—An enzyme that helps digest the lactose in milk.

LACTATION—Secretion of milk by the mammary gland.

LACTOSE—A sugar found naturally in milk.

LACTOSE INTOLERANCE—The inability to properly assimilate (*see* Assimilation) milk due to lack of lactase (*see* Lactase) enzyme.

LEGUME—Any of a large family of herbs, shrubs and trees including peas and beans, with fruit growing in a pod.

LOW BLOOD SUGAR (Hypoglycemia)—An abnormally low level of glucose (*see* Glucose) in the blood.

MALNUTRITION—Poor nourishment resulting from insufficient food or improper diet.

MARGARINE—A spread or cooking fat made of refined vegetable oils.

METABOLISM—The chemical and physical process going on in living organisms in which food is assimilated and built into body cells.

METABOLITE—Any substance taking part in the chemical process of living cells and organisms.

METHYL XANTHINE—A family of chemicals including caffeine. A stimulant to the central nervous system. Also found in tea, cocoa, and chocolate.

NUTRITION—The process of taking in and assimilating food for promoting growth and replacing worn or injured tissue.

OXIDATION—The union of a substance with oxygen.

PASTEURIZATION—Heating liquid to a prescribed temperature for a specified period of time to check the activity and fermentation of bacteria.

PECTIN—The breakdown of plant tissue that holds cell walls together. The richest source is in apples.

PROSTAGLANDINS—A hormone produced in cells for minute by minute activity as needed.

SATURATED—That which has absorbed all that can be taken up. (Fat molecule filled to capacity with hydrogen atoms.) Saturated fat is usually solid at room temperature.

SESAME SEEDS (PROTEIN-AIDE BRAND)—Sesame seeds exclusively hulled without chemicals. A unique protein complementary food for vegetarian diets.

ULTRAPASTEURIZED—Heating a product to more than 200°F to increase shelf life (as ultrapasteurized milk or ultrapasteurized cream).

UNSATURATED—A fat in liquid state that can combine with more hydrogen; a compound in which some element possesses the capacity of combining further with another element.

INDEX